T0123694

What They Said about *The Art of Mackin'*

"Nasheed's manual 'is the first "how-to" book that teaches men how to become "players" and "macks" '—hip-hop versions of the old-fashioned cad—'and how to use "pimp game" as a form of manipulation (not deceit) in order to get what they want from women.' What kind of women? Nasheed breaks them down: there's the Top-Notch Sista ('when dealing with a top-notch sista, brothers have to really come correct'); the Middle-Class Girl; the Hoodrat; and the Chickenhead (a classification Nasheed further splits into the Low-Budget and the Straight-Up Hoochie Chickenhead; to spot the latter, be on the lookout for gold teeth and lips that are 'purple from smoking weed'). To woo these women, Nasheed recommends that men model themselves on (a) the neighborhood pimp, and (b) Bill Clinton. Regarding (a) he writes: 'One has to admit that it takes some serious game for a brother to have a stable of women "breakin' him off cheddar" on the regular.' (Cheddar, by the way, means money.) As to (b), Nasheed notes that when Clinton's dalliance with Monica Lewinsky went public, 'he went on television and started spitting game.' And his game was so tight, his popularity rating with the public went *up*. Now, if that is not a mack, I don't know what is.' "
—*The New York Times Book Review*

"An excellent book."
—Big Boy, Power 106, Los Angeles

"I dove headlong into *Mackin'* . . . The thinking man's practical guide to dating, and the thinking woman's secret weapon for defusing and short circuiting would-be players and micro-pimps. Equal parts political science, common sense, and wry observation, the book defines the art of macking with a cold, honest, Machiavellian precision. Macking is less about exploitation than about going after what you want. It is the art of inequitable exchange, where both parties are satisfied with their portion. *Mackin'* is hard on would-be macks, admonishing men to control their sexual needs and not 'lie on they dick.' He discourages macking beyond your means, and lets it be known that 'moochin' don't make you no mack.' Game respects game, and Nasheed recognizes that macking is the gift of rhetoric more than anything. He drops dap when he sees a true master at work. *Mackin'* is not for the Pierre Delacroix, milk-sopped-typa bruthas, lyalanites or Oprahphiles in need of a hug. Like Sun Tzu's *Art of War*, *Mackin'* dispenses advice and strategem that can be applied to any of life's moral quandaries, from the bedroom to the boardroom."
—Jimi Izrael

"A much needed book."
—*The Source*

"A true expert on mackin'."
—Jenny Jones

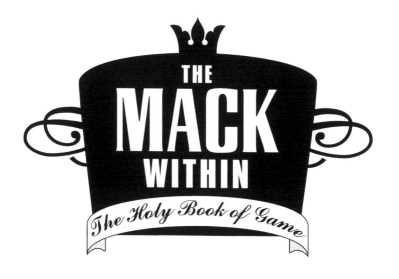

Tariq "King Flex" Nasheed

RIVERHEAD FREESTYLE
NEW YORK

THE BERKLEY PUBLISHING GROUP
Published by the Penguin Group
Penguin Group (USA) Inc.
375 Hudson Street, New York, New York 10014, USA
Penguin Group (Canada), 90 Eglinton Avenue East, Suite 700, Toronto, Ontario M4P 2Y3, Canada
(a division of Pearson Penguin Canada Inc.)
Penguin Books Ltd., 80 Strand, London WC2R 0RL, England
Penguin Group Ireland, 25 St. Stephen's Green, Dublin 2, Ireland (a division of Penguin Books Ltd.)
Penguin Group (Australia), 250 Camberwell Road, Camberwell, Victoria 3124, Australia
(a division of Pearson Australia Group Pty. Ltd.)
Penguin Books India Pvt. Ltd., 11 Community Centre, Panchsheel Park, New Delhi—110 017, India
Penguin Group (NZ), Cnr. Airborne and Rosedale Roads, Albany, Auckland 1310, New Zealand
(a division of Pearson New Zealand Ltd.)
Penguin Books (South Africa) (Pty.) Ltd., 24 Sturdee Avenue, Rosebank, Johannesburg 2196,
South Africa

Penguin Books Ltd., Registered Offices: 80 Strand, London WC2R 0RL, England

Copyright © 2005 by Tariq Nasheed
Cover design by Benjamin Gibson
Cover photographs by Kevin Stagger
Cover models: Erin Green and Mori
Photo stylist: Tasha Monica Carter for TMC Fashion Co.
Book design by Tiffany Estreicher

First Riverhead Freestyle trade paperback edition: October 2005

Library of Congress Cataloging-in-Publication Data

Nasheed, Tariq
        The mack within / Tariq "King Flex" Nasheed.
            p.   cm.
        Additional title information on dust jacket: the holy book of game.
        ISBN 978-1-59448-179-6
        1. Dating (Social customs)—United States.   2. Man-woman relationships—United States.
    3. African Americans—Sexual behavior.   4. African Americans—Social life and customs.
    5. Control (Psychology)   I. Title.

    HQ801.N3635   2005
    646.7'7'08996073—dc22

2005048022

147468846

IN THE WORDS OF A MACK . . .

Call Girl: A female who works through an agency or escort service, dealing with high-paying tricks.

Captain Save-a-Ho: A man who tries to earn the attention and affection of women by offering them support (often financial). This term derives from the hip-hop song "Captain Save-a-Ho" by E-40.

Chickenhead: A female who is content to live in substandard conditions. A female with no game who doesn't want to achieve higher learning.

Dime: A female who is considered a ten out of ten based on physical beauty.

Gigolo: A man who offers sexual gratification and companionship to square women in exchange for financial benefits.

Hoochie: A female who overly accentuates her looks to the point of gaudiness.

Hoodrat: A female who lives in a low-income, inner-city area.

Hustler: A person who utilizes a specific gift, trade, or skill to make money.

Mack: A man who is motivated by knowledge and power and who understands that once he *achieves* knowledge and power and applies some hustle to his game, females and money will come automatically.

Pimp: A man who is financially motivated. A man who serves as a companion, boss, and mentor to working women in the game (i.e., strippers, hookers, call girls, etc.).

Player: A man who has tailored his verbal skills in order to get the largest number of potential sex partners. A man who is sexually motivated.

Pussy-whipped: What a man is said to be when he has taken on a submissive, subservient position with a female in order to maintain sexual favors.

Slut: A female whose primary desire is to receive sexual gratification from a number of different people.

Square: A person who is not in the game and not a professional hustler. A person with a nine-to-five job.

Stank: A female who provides sexual gratification for menial items (such as food, beer, weed, etc.).

Stella: An older female who overtly flirts with a number of younger men in order to see if she is still sexually desirable. From the book and movie *How Stella Got Her Groove Back*.

Trick: A man who pays for sexual gratification.

KING FLEX'S TEN COMMANDMENTS OF MACKIN'

1. Mackin' is 20 percent talk, 80 percent attitude.

If your game and your gear are tight enough, you can pull females without saying anything at all.

2. There are only two ways to handle any relationship situation: Like a trick, or like a mack.

When a relationship problem arises, a man is either going to mack up, or trick off. You're either going to be a player or a payer. Always be a mack.

3. To be a true mack, you must have integrity.

To be a mack is to be a boss. And in order to be a leader, you must be worthy of being followed.

4. Always qualify your females before you start mackin'.

Mackin' to a female who isn't qualified to receive good game is like speaking Chinese to a Mexican. No matter how tight your game is, she simply won't understand.

5. Respect the rules of the game.

The mackin' game, on a street level, is the only hustle with its own set of rules. Anyone can be a drug dealer. Anyone can be a car-jacker. But you must abide by certain rules to be a successful mack.

6. A mack must be tactful.

A mack's game should always be appropriate to the situation. Don't be overly energetic when you should be low-key, and vice-versa. Remember that there is a time and place for everything.

7. A true mack must always have options.

You should always be in a position where you can recruit and dismiss (also known as "cop and blow") females at whim. The day your females see that you have run out of options is the day you lose.

8. Never follow your woman.

It's ok to get input from your woman. It's even ok to get knowledge from your woman. But the minute you put your woman in a position of leadership over you, she will lose respect for you. Never let your woman determine your role in the relationship. It's your job as a mack to set your own agenda.

9. A mack must constantly upgrade his game and reinvent himself.

Familiarity breeds contempt. You must always keep your females in suspense, never knowing what you will do next. A true mack must always have new tricks up his sleeve.

10. Require your females to bring more to the table than just sexual gratification.

If you don't require your lady to bring any real assets to the table, she will assume that her sexual gratification is an asset, thus putting you in the position of a trick. You must let women know that sex is so readily available to you that it has no value.

CONTENTS

INTRODUCTION

Rolling Stone recently sent a reporter who was a total square out here to Los Angeles to do a feature story on me. He was looking for insight into my lifestyle, my success, and the whole mack subculture of the streets, but he also wanted to test me to see if I lived up to my reputation of being able to turn any man into a mack. That's right, this dude wanted to hang with me for a week to see if I could give him a Mack Makeover.

Now when I say this reporter was square, I mean he was a *total* square. It's easy for me to teach people in the young, urban demographic, because most of them are at least somewhat familiar with the game. But here I was dealing with a square, middle-aged white guy who looked like an insurance salesman. He looked like the adult version of Harry Potter.

And it was now my job to turn Clark Kent into Supermack.

The first thing I needed to do was to get his tools together. I took him to one of my favorite clothing spots to get him some new

gear. The whole mackin' world was so new to him that he was literally trembling with nervousness as he was trying on his new
clothes.

Next, we rolled around town while I broke the game down to
him. I gave him the basics of the mackin' game, and he was soaking it
all up like a sponge. The reporter told me that he had been divorced
for about four years after twenty years of marriage. He admitted that
he knew absolutely nothing about the current dating scene, let alone
how to approach a woman. So I schooled him on the rules of the
game, and later on that night, we set out to go to the club. This club
was one of the hottest spots in Los Angeles. I knew that a lot of top-
notch females liked to hang there, so I brought some of my best mack
partners with us.

Now I will admit, it did look kind of odd to have five young
black guys and one middle-aged white guy hanging out at the club
together. We told the reporter that people are going to think that
he is our probation officer. But the vibe was cool, and he realized
that he was in good hands with us. In the club, the reporter does
everything that I tell him to do. He carries himself the way I tell
him. And to his surprise, females were coming up to *him* starting
conversations. Throughout the night, we saw the reporter interacting with different females, exchanging numbers, the whole nine.
He was shocked to see that females there were so receptive to him.
He didn't know he had it in him to pull women like that. He told
me that he was now a believer. All I did was tap into his mack
within.

The same game that I shared with that *Rolling Stone* reporter is
what I'm going to share with you in this book. And if the sprinkle
of game I laced that reporter with could upgrade his game that

dramatically, just imagine what a whole book of the game can do for you.

The Mack Within is a book designed to help men live up to their full mack potential. Let's face it: Most men would love to have the game and confidence to get not only any type of female he wants, but also to achieve any goal he wants to in life. And despite the macho, "I-don't-need-no-help" facade that many men hide behind, the reality is, a lot of guys are frustrated from not getting the results they really want out of dating.

The first thing a potential mack has to understand is that the mackin' game isn't about ego or emotions. It's about logic. You have to mack from your mind, not from your heart. If you are the type of cat who is emotionally driven, and you insist on getting your heart involved with every female you meet, this book isn't for you. If you are one of those masochistic guys who secretly enjoys being played like a sucker by females, this book isn't for you. If you are one of those guys who is proud to be a "hopeless romantic," just put down this book and go pick up *The Best of Lionel Richie*.

This book is for the guys who seriously want to put the mack down. Let me ask you:

- Are you tired of being Mr. Nice Guy and getting nowhere with females?

- Are you tired of waiting until you become a successful rapper or athlete before you can get the type of woman you really want?

- Are you tired of tricking off drinks at clubs, just so women will talk to you?

- Are you tired of settling for second- and third-rate females, wishing you could get with females that look like the ones in music videos?

- Are you tired of being sexually manipulated by females?

- Are you tired of having to spend excessive amounts of money on females just to have them in your company?

If you answered "yes" to any of these questions, this book is for you.

Before you can soak up all the game in this book, you must disregard everything that you have been taught about man/woman relationships. Forget everything you were taught in the square world. This book is going to give you insight straight from the street world. You will learn that the rules regarding man/woman relationships on a street level can be directly applied to relationships in the square world.

This book will also give you important mackin' pointers on topics like:

- **How soon to call a female after you meet her**

- **How much money to spend on a first date**

- **How to mack to females at malls, bus stops, and other common spots**

- **Which females you should avoid**

- **How to get females to cater to your every need**

With *The Mack Within*, I'm not trying to turn men into something they are not. There are different types of macks, and different levels of mackin'. I just want to bring men to a level of mackin' that is comfortable for them and fits their individual desires.

There are a lot of guys out there who have the raw materials for being a true mack, but they don't know how to channel their energy. I remember when Kobe Bryant first got into the NBA. Everyone knew he was a good player, but he and his team weren't winning games. Kobe was infamous for hogging the ball and was perceived as a self-centered player. He was a good basketball player, but he wasn't a good *game* player. So when Phil Jackson came into the picture, he showed Kobe how to hone his talents, and to utilize his skills correctly to become a *team* player. And that was when Kobe started to win championships. I'll help you tap into your mack within and help you develop your raw mackin' skills so you can start winning in the dating game. You can look at me as the Phil Jackson of mackin'.

The Mack Within isn't a book on how to get over on women, or how to deceive women. The word *mack* has become an almost misogynistic term in our society today. This book will also help clear up a lot of those myths and misconceptions about the true essence of what a mack really is. When you tap into the mack within, you will learn to find that balance and inner peace with yourself.

Too many men are coochie-whipped in our society. This is frustrating to both men and women, because women eventually become frustrated with men they can dominate and control sexually. A lot of men are under the false impression that they are running the show in their relationships. And the worst part of being coochie-whipped is not knowing that you are.

Here are a few signs that you are coochie-whipped, and you need to soak up this game:

- **If you and your lady go out wearing matching outfits**

- **If your lady sends you to the store to get her feminine products**

- **If your lady makes you hold her purse at the mall**

- **If you had to hide this book from your lady**

If any of these things apply to you, it's time to learn how to tap into the mack within.

1

THE MACK IN YOU

Every man has the potential to be a mack. It's as simple as that. Every man. Yes, that means you, too. The question is, to what degree? There are first-degree macks, second-degree macks, and third-degree macks. Let me break it down for you.

First-Degree Macks

When a man becomes sexually active for the first time, he automatically becomes a first-degree mack. And after he gets his first taste of sex, he wants to know two things and two things only: how to get more women, and how to get *better* women. And in the mind of most first-degree macks, more *is* better.

So the first-degree mack spends most of his time trying to figure out how to get more and better women. Even if the first-degree mack settles for a subpar female, he still has secret desires to have better.

Which brings us to . . .

Second-Degree Macks

Second-degree macks are guys who are more experienced and who have figured out effective techniques for getting women. The second-degree mack's primary focus in life is to get as many notches on his belt—that is, sexual partners—as possible. These guys are commonly known as "players."

Second-degree mack is the highest level of mackin' that the average man will reach in his life. This is because the average man has been taught to value sex over everything else. (More on that topic later.)

Third-Degree Macks

Third-degree macks have been through their player stage and have decided to upgrade their game. Third-degree macks understand that when it comes to females, it's all about *quality* instead of *quantity*. The third-degree mack knows why one top-notch female is better than twenty chickenheads.

This book will get you to the third-degree level of mackin'. And once you have reached the third-degree level of mackin', you have truly tapped into the mack within.

The Foundation of a True Mack

What you must first understand about the game is that **mackin' starts in the mind**. It doesn't start when you get an NBA contract. It doesn't start when you get a record deal. It doesn't start when you buy some new rims, a Rolex, or an Escalade.

If you need material things to make you feel like a mack, what will happen if you lose those things? You won't feel like a mack anymore. Let's say you get women based on what your car looks like. If your car were to be repossessed or put in the shop, you wouldn't get women anymore. Or, let's say you get women strictly because you have a hit song on the charts at the moment. What's going to happen when you don't have any more hits? That's right, no more women. The same thing that happened to Billy Ocean, Christopher Williams, Rico Suave, and the cats who made "Whoomp There It Is." No more females are sweating them.

This is why it's important to focus on having *game*. You can lose all of your superficial material possessions, but game can never be taken away from you. This is why you must understand that mackin' starts in the mind. Mackin' is all about how you view yourself. Because the way you see yourself in your own mind is the way others will eventually see you, too.

If you see yourself as a sucker, or as insecure, others will see you that way, too. But if you see yourself as a boss player, people will treat you like one.

Confidence Is a Must

The most important tool for a potential mack is self-confidence. When you have confidence, you look like a winner. And everyone, fine women included, loves to be around a winner.

When you have confidence, it shows not only in your words, but in your nonverbal cues, as well. People always come up to me asking for clever pick-up lines to use on women. And I tell them, it's not about pick-up lines. It's about having confidence. I can tell some guys what to say verbatim, but if they don't have the confidence to back up those words, they are going to get shut down by females anyway.

When you have the confidence to back up your words, you can say just about anything to a female and look fly. You can walk up to a female and tell her that her weave is out of place, and she will still be feeling you. Remember, it's not what you say, but how you say it.

To Be a Mack, You Must Have Your Priorities Straight

The top four things aspiring macks are insecure about:

1. Their occupations
2. Their cars
3. Their cribs
4. Their looks

I always get e-mails from guys saying things like, "*Yo, King Flex, I don't have my own place, I don't have a job, and I don't have a car.*

So what's the best way for me to get females under my circumstances?"

I tell these guys to get their priorities in order, and work on areas where they are lacking that make them insecure before stepping into the mackin' arena. If you are trying to mack on a female and you have things that you are insecure about, you may find yourself lacking confidence and focusing on whether or not the female is going to find out about them, rather than on the quality of your game. You can't be 100 percent on-point with your game if you are wondering what a female will think of you when she finds out you live with your mom. Your game can't be up to par if you are wondering what she'll think if you pull up to her crib in a bucket.

So this is why it's important for a potential mack to not try to mask or hide his shortcomings, but to rectify them. A playa must focus on stackin' his paper first. A playa must focus on increasing his game first. If you have issues with being out of shape, you must first focus on working out. Because guess what? After you get your game together, after you stack your paper, after you get your hustle on, those same females are still going to be there.

Top Five Fabrics True Macks Like to Wear

1. Mink
2. Silk
3. Leather
4. Suede
5. Chinchilla

Top Five Fabrics Macks Do Not Wear

1. Lace
2. Macramé
3. Nylon
4. Corduroy
5. Pleather

2

WHAT KIND OF MACK ARE YOU?

In order for a man to reach true mackdom, he has to understand what type of man he is. He must also understand where his level of game is, as well. Before a man can understand the psychological and social makeup of different types of women, he has to be able to correctly analyze himself. This way he can correctly diagnose his strengths and deficiencies, and therefore make the correct adjustments and upgrades if need be. In this chapter I will place men in eight different categories. I will refer to these men as the *eight S's.*

They are:

1. The Smooth Brother
2. The Serious Brother
3. The Sensitive Simp
4. The Save-a-Ho Brother
5. The Sassy Brother
6. The Scavenger

7. The Super Thug
8. The Scrub

Here's the breakdown:

The Smooth Brother

The Smooth Brother is the cat who has the gift of gab. He knows what to say and how to say it when it comes to spitting game at females. Smooth Brothers are very laid back and mellow with their game, and they know how to talk their way out of certain predicaments with women (especially in cases of infidelity).

This Smooth Brother usually has one main lady and several females on the side. He also takes pride in being able to juggle a number of women without any one of them finding out about another.

Positive Aspects of the Smooth Brother

The positive thing about Smooth Brothers is that many of them are very charismatic and suave. Many Smooth Brothers also know how to intrigue women by using their personality and charm. Many of these guys are snappy dressers and they know not to be too over-the-top with their gear. Many Smooth Brothers also know how to turn women on with words, which is a major requirement for being a true mack.

Negative Aspects of the Smooth Brother

On the negative side, many Smooth Brothers are somewhat deceitful in the way they deal with women. Many of these guys are habitual liars, and they get a thrill from being able to get away with their most outrageous lies.

One of the rules of the mackin' game is that you have to play it fair. But many Smooth Brothers have a take-no-prisoners attitude when it comes to dealing with women. They will live a lie as long as they can get away with it. They revel in deceit. And once the women they deal with become aware of the deceptive Smooth Brother's lies, these women will ultimately lose respect for them. A true mack must maintain a level of respect from his women at all times.

The Smooth Brother's Game

The Smooth Brother usually steps to women in a very laid-back manner. He has learned how to master the art of *reaction*. He knows how to make smooth and clever responses to everything a female says to him. Females are usually impressed by his verbal spontaneity and quick wit. The effortlessness of his on-point responses during conversation is usually what lures women in.

The Serious Brother

The Serious Brother is usually the no-nonsense, suit-and-tie professional guy who does things by the book. The Serious Brother is usually well-disciplined and well-educated, and in many cases he is very financially stable. Many Serious Brothers have extensive college or military backgrounds, and they take great pride in their academic achievements.

Positive Aspects of the Serious Brother

The positive thing about Serious Brothers is that they have no time for games or half-assing. Serious Brothers are very thorough when it comes to taking care of business. They earn the respect and trust of those around them. Many women find Serious Brothers desirable because these guys are usually intelligent, dependable, and they provide a sense of security. And women consider this as marriage material in a man.

Negative Aspects of the Serious Brother

On the flip side of the Serious Brother, many of these guys are considered assholes. Because many of the Serious Brothers are well-educated and financially stable, they sometimes tend to have a holier-than-thou attitude. Sometimes these cats are so serious, they forget that they need to loosen up and have fun every once in a while. Some of the Serious Brothers possess this know-it-all attitude that can start weighing on people's nerves after a while. And even though women like a man who is well-educated and who knows how to handle business, women also like a man who can have a little fun every now and then.

The Serious Brother's Game

The Serious Brother likes to use his credentials to impress the women he steps to. He likes to brag about his college and academic degrees, his worldly travels, and basically his knowledge of the finer things in life. This can work two ways. It can make him look intelligent. Or it could make him appear as if he's belittling the females he's trying to get with. When you are trying to flex your knowledge, you have to be very subtle about it. Never bring up a topic that you just happen to be knowledgeable about out of the blue. I knew one Serious Brother who would get around females and start talking about computers. He thought showing his extensive knowledge would impress females, but the way he did it made him look like an ass. Only flex your academic knowledge around females if the conversation happens to casually shift to that subject matter or if the female brings up the subject.

The Sensitive Simp

The Sensitive Simp is the type of cat who loves to pamper women and cater to their every need. This is the type of guy who likes to bring flowers and candy to a female on a first date. These guys also like to do things like send poems to women, send females cute little e-mails all day, and stand outside a woman's window with a guitar, serenading her with love songs. Many of the Sensitive Simps grew up in households where women were the dominant force, so they grow up thinking that being submissive to women is the natural order of things.

Many of these guys have somewhat of a masochistic desire to cater to women. The more they get dissed by women, the more they have an urge to cater to them. These guys take the "kill them with kindness" mentality to an extreme level. The Sensitive Simp feels that if he caters to women and treats them nicely, eventually he will win them over.

Positive aspects of the Sensitive Simp

There are times when a man needs to show some sensitivity when dealing with women. There are special occasions (such as Christmas, Valentine's Day, birthdays, anniversaries, etc.) when a man should be somewhat romantic to a female. As long as you are showing appreciation for a female based on the things she has done for you, there is nothing wrong with showing your sensitive side every now and then. Just don't start simpin' right out the gate.

Negative Aspects of the Sensitive Simp

The negative thing about Sensitive Simps is that many of them come across like wimpy mama's boys who are desperate for female affection. And this usually turns women completely off. Many of these men are insecure, and women can sense this. Women like men who are somewhat of a challenge. And when a man goes out of his way to cater to a woman, by chasing her and rolling out the red carpet for her too much and too soon, this takes away from the challenge.

Women might *claim* they like the Keith Sweat, Michael Bolton, or Brian McKnight type of romance from a guy, but they say this because it's the politically correct thing to say. Most women will claim they like a certain type of guy, but then they will turn around and date the complete opposite of what they claim to like. The problem with the Sensitive Simp is that he actually believes women when they claim they want a sensitive man. True macks know better than to fall for the "I really want a nice, sensitive guy" script.

The Sensitive Simp's Game

The Sensitive Simp usually steps to women with extreme gratitude. He likes to show a female how appreciative he is that she would take time out of her life to show him any form of attention. The Sensitive Simp steps to women by kissing ass right out the gate. He likes to shower them with compliments and praise. And the Sensitive Simp will get around a woman and agree with everything she says. He does this because he doesn't want to do anything to jeopardize his chances of staying on a female's good side.

The Save-a-Ho Brother

The Save-a-Ho Brother (a term that comes from the '90s rap song "Captain Save-a-Ho" by E-40) is a guy who tries to portray himself as a knight in shining armor to women. The Save-a-Ho Brother likes to seek out damsels in distress or women who are in need of some sort of financial assistance. These men like to offer their financial assistance to women because this is the only way they feel that they can get their foot in the door.

Save-a-Ho Brothers are the type of guys who like to brag about how much they could do for a woman financially if she were with him instead of her current man. And these are the type of guys who like to go to titty bars and try to square up strippers. Many of these cats feel that if all the women out there took the time to get to know them, they could turn any ho into a housewife.

Positive Aspects of the Save-a-Ho Brother

There's nothing wrong with financially helping out a female, *as long as you know for sure she would do the same for you*. If a female has brought something to the table for you, it's perfectly fine to help her out every once in a while. But as a mack, you need to "spit game and holla, before you spend change and dollas." Don't spend money on a female in hopes of trying to impress her or win her over. One other good thing about the Save-a-Ho Brother in particular is that they provide females with the money and material items to spend on true macks like us.

Negative Aspects of the Save-a-Ho Brother

Save-a-Ho Brothers use money and the promise of financial gain to lure women in, because they erroneously believe that women would never bite the hand that feeds them. Nothing could be further from the truth. Save-a-Ho Brothers are basic tricks. And women will accept tricks, but deep down, they do not *respect* tricks.

Plus, many women resent the feeling of having to owe something to the Save-a-Ho Brother in return for him doing favors for them. Eventually that feeling of resentment turns into utter contempt. This is because people generally hate to feel obligated or indebted to other people.

For example, do you ever notice how people act toward credit-card collection agencies? Credit-card companies basically front people money. And people are generally more than happy to spend that money. But when it comes time to pay that money back, people start acting funky as hell. People start ducking and dodging, trying to avoid the credit-card collectors. And some people actually get *offended* that the credit-card companies want their money back. This is the same feeling that women have toward Save-a-Ho Brothers. Women hate the feeling of having to "owe ass" to a guy just because he keeps volunteering to help her pay her utility bills.

The Save-a-Ho Brother's Game

The Save-a-Ho Brother usually steps to women with his credit card in his hand. His game is to simply use money to try to impress females. He is the kind of guy who will buy drinks for a girl and all of her friends at the club. He uses money to compensate for his lack of game. The Save-a-Ho Brother will step to females and offer them trips to the mall and other types of shopping sprees. If a female has kids, he will offer to take them to Chuck E. Cheese's. His game is to make the female become dependent on him. He feels that if a woman is financially dependent on him, he is in control.

The Sassy Brother

"Sassy" is a term for men that is synonymous with being "metrosexual." A Sassy Brother isn't necessarily gay, but the clothes he wears tend to make people think that he's "suspect." The Sassy Brother is the male equivalent of a hoochie, dressing to get attention. These are the Eric Benet– or Lenny Kravitz–type cats who you see in the club wearing things like see-through shirts, chokers, tongue rings, lace, toe rings, or ankle bracelets. Basically, Sassy Brothers like to wear the total opposite of what a true mack would wear.

Positive Aspects of the Sassy Brother

The one good thing about the Sassy Brother is that he does take pride in the way he looks. Many guys will just throw on anything they've got lying around and go out to the club. But the Sassy Brother takes his time and tries to coordinate his gear.

Negative Aspects of the Sassy Brother

Even though the Sassy Brother does put thought into coordinating his attire, he sometimes overdoes it. A true mack has to be very careful when he is coordinating his gear. Because one wrong accessory can make a perfectly fly outfit look sassy. You can have on a mackish, all-black Armani suit, but if you put on a pair of pink boots with it, guess what? Your ass is sassy.

The Sassy Brother's Game

Most men understand that when women dress sexy or skimpy they will attract men. But Sassy Brothers think that if *they* dress sexy or skimpy, they will impress *women,* as well. Sassy Brothers will step to women with their shirts open one button too many. They will try to wear outfits that show off their abs. They will wear open-toed shoes, etc. These guys will put on their sassy gear, post up, and wait for females to compliment them on their attire.

The Scavenger

A scavenger, by definition, is someone who accepts leftovers and things that are undesirable. And there are guys out there who have this mentality when it comes to dating. In every group of guys, there is always at least *one* Scavenger. We all have that one homeboy who will bang *anything*. And if you can't figure out who that homeboy is in your group of friends, it's probably *you*.

Positive Aspects of the Scavenger

The one good thing about the Scavenger is that if a group of guys meets a group of girls, and one of the girls is a duck, you could hook up your Scavenger homeboy with her. Whenever you meet a group of women, the least attractive ones (usually the ones no other guys will talk to) always try to throw salt in your game. So it's always good to have a Scavenger partner with you to intercept any cock-blocking.

Even in the wild, scavengers (such as hyenas and vultures, etc.) are essential to nature because they dispose of waste and bring balance to the ecosystem. And if it weren't for Scavenger brothers, no one would be available to occupy all the chickenheads and hoodrats who slip through the cracks.

Negative Aspects of the Scavenger

The one downside of having a Scavenger homeboy is that oftentimes he will drag a "dead carcass" into your circle. Scavengers will bring a chickenhead and all of her chickenhead friends around you and your partners. And this makes your clique look bad. So in some instances, you have to keep the Scavenger in your inner circle at arm's length, because a true mack's game is often judged on the quality of females he can attract. And if you have a gang of chickenheads hanging around your crew, it shows a deficiency in your game.

The Scavenger's Game

The Scavenger's game is simple: He usually steps to women in the clubs that nobody else wants. He keeps his standards extremely low so that his rate of rejection is minimal. Also, the Scavenger is the master of parking-lot pimpin'. Scavengers like to hang around outside of clubs until they close for the night so they can pick up the strays. True macks try not to stay at clubs until they close, because the quality of women who hang around parking lots of clubs are usually not up to par. Quality women like to show up to the club late, and leave the club early. They usually have to get up the next morning to do something productive. But low-budget women will literally stay at the club all night and stick around afterward. And the Scavengers will be right there to keep them company.

The Super Thug

The Super Thug is that in-and-out-of-jail brother who only thinks in terms of his survival. These are the gangsta-type cats who don't play by anyone's rules, and they are down to do whatever. These are the guys who are involved with carjackings, stickups, and dope-dealing. Super Thugs have no sense of morality; therefore they have no remorse for the people they get over on. Now, don't confuse the Super Thug with the wannabe thug who only pretends to be gangsta because now it's the hip thing to do. Super Thugs are those three-strikes, always-on-parole brothers who come from families three generations deep in the ghetto.

Positive Aspects of the Super Thug

Because of their overly macho, self-assured attitude, many females find Super Thugs sexually enticing, in a primal sort of way. Many females gleefully confess that thug brothers "know how to hit it rough." Another thing about the Super Thug is that he always has "the hook-up" on something. Whatever you need, these cats can always get it for you at a discounted rate. Super Thugs always have the hook-up on cars, clothes, jewelry, DVD players, etc. We all know that *one* brother who can get a thirty-inch, flat-screen color TV for $80. If you ever want to keep an ear to the street, the Super Thug is your go-to guy.

Negative Aspects of the Super Thug

The bad thing about many Super Thugs is that they really don't have any long-term lucrative hustle. Most of these guys have a smash-and-grab mentality. That's the difference between a *hustler* and a *scam artist*. A hustler tries to make continuous, long-term benefits with the least amount of risk. But with the scam artists, the negative consequences and penalties outweigh the rewards. A hustler will set up shop, hire the right people, *bribe* the right people, operate under the radar, and stack paper over a long period of time.

A scam artist will rob a liquor store for $100, get caught, and do twenty years in prison. Unfortunately, many Super Thugs have this self-defeating mentality.

The Super Thug's Game

Super Thugs usually step to ghetto girls and other hoodrats who live in their neighborhoods. Super Thugs like to date women they can smoke weed with and get drunk with. So their game is to seek out women who like to get high, and chickenheads usually fit the bill. Another reason why ghetto girls are more susceptible to the Super Thug's game is because many females from the hood grew up with no strong male figure in their lives, so they have no real perception of what true manhood is. Therefore, they assume that the overly macho demeanor of the Super Thug is a true representation of a real man.

The Scrub

The Scrub is the consummate underachiever who never really has anything going for himself. This is the kind of guy who lives with his mother until he's in his thirties. The Scrub is the eternal teenager who never wants to grow up. These are the type of guys who sit around the house all day smoking weed and playing Xbox. Scrubs usually have very low expectations in life. Their primary focus is when the new Jordans are coming out and what type of rims they should put on their '82 Oldsmobile Cutlass Supreme.

Positive Aspects of the Scrub

The good thing about Scrubs is that they make excellent flunkies. Scrubs are natural followers. So if you need someone to take on menial, insignificant tasks for you, the Scrub can always be counted on. Even though most Scrubs don't work full-time jobs, it is not too hard to get one to do a small task for you. All they need to do is make enough money to get their next bag of weed and they will be straight. Another thing about Scrubs is that many of them have no problem putting their bid in when it comes to women. If you go to a club, the brokest Scrub in the room will be the first one up in a female's face, trying to kick game. Many Scrubs feel that since they have no crib of their own, no job, no car, and no real money to speak of, they really have nothing else to lose by spitting game at all the females.

Negative Aspects of the Scrub

Many Scrubs have negative, "broke" energy. And if you hang around slackers long enough, that loser energy can rub off on you. Many Scrubs are haters, as well. Scrubs hate seeing other brothers doing better than them. This is especially true if you started out in the same boat as the Scrub, but you upgraded your game. When you become more prosperous in life than your Scrub counterpart, this reinforces the loser self-image the Scrub has of himself. So in order for this Scrub to cope with his shortcomings, he has to project his negative feelings onto you.

The Scrub's Game

The Scrub steps to women using the slot-machine technique. He simply talks to every female he sees until he hits the jackpot. Basically, his game depends on luck. The Scrub has no problem being rejected by a thousand women, as long as he gets some play from one of them. His game is based on numbers and averages. Also, Scrubs love to hang around guys who are more financially stable or whose game is tighter than theirs. Scrubs like to floss in their homeboys' cars. Scrubs like to take females to their homeboys' cribs. Scrubs like to catch all of their homeboys' leftover females. Another game that the Scrubs have is the baby-daddy hustle. Scrubs like to have children by as many women as possible (usually hoodrats), so they can live off of them.

What Type of Man Makes the Best Mack?

You are probably wondering which one of these eight S's has the most true mack potential. The answer isn't so simple. All of the eight S's have their own brand of game, but in order for a man to reach the pinnacle of true mackdom, he has to be a psychological shape-shifter. He has to be able to adopt many different personality traits. He has to become what I call an **Urban Renaissance Man**. And in order to be an Urban Renaissance Man, you have to incorporate all of the positive aspects of the eight S's.

You have to be charismatic like the **Smooth Brother**. You have to be able to handle your financial business like the **Serious Brother**. You have to be somewhat compassionate at times, like the

Sensitive Simp. You have to be able to provide for the right female (who will provide for you in return) like the **Save-a-Ho Brother**. You have to be somewhat fashion-conscious like the **Sassy Brother**. You have to be able to work as a team with other players in your entourage, like the **Scavenger**. You have to be able to spit game at a number of females, like the **Scrub**. And when it gets down to it, you have to be able to get with a female and tap that ass gangster-style, like the **Super Thug**.

Top Five Macks in Hollywood

1. Denzel Washington
2. Warren Beatty
3. Jack Nicholson
4. George Clooney
5. Bob Barker

3

A MACK MUST VALUE HIMSELF

To be a true mack, you must first disregard everything your mother ever told you about dating and relationships. We are currently living in a time where many of us grow up without fathers in the household. As a result, we have a generation of men getting into relationships guided only by advice from a female point of view. This is part of why many men are disillusioned by and bitter about dating—they don't have father figures to share time-tested wisdom with them.

Now, I'm not trying to throw salt on the single mothers out there. I honestly believe that many single mothers mean well when they try to teach their sons about how to interact with females. But many of these single mothers give their sons the rose-colored-glasses point of view on dating, instead of the real story. And subsequently, many young men are misinformed about how to deal with women.

How Mothers Program Their Sons to Be Tricks and Their Daughters to Be Hos

Even though there are exceptions to this theory, most mothers out there (especially single mothers) teach their sons to be tricks, even though mackin' is the natural instinct for men. As I've said, every man has a mack within. Every heterosexual man wants a *variety* of women or the *best* women. But many are brainwashed from a young age by their mothers, sometimes subtly and sometimes blatantly, to be tricks.

It starts off with mothers telling their sons that they should treat *all* women as special. Boys are taught that they should respect all women, that *all* women are a prize. Boys are taught to pull out chairs for women, open car doors for women, spread their coats over puddles for women, etc. Basically, boys are taught that anyone with a vagina should be highly valued. This programs men to worship female sexuality. Men are given no other reason for the necessity of their giving indiscriminate respect and value to females other than the fact that they have different sexual organs.

The reality is that men should *not* be taught to respect all women, because not *all* women are worthy of respect, just as not *all* men are worthy of respect. Respect is not a given. It is something you *earn*. And there are women and men alike who don't even respect themselves, so why should anyone be obligated to respect them simply based on their gender?

Many mothers who misinform their sons know the whole truth, but don't want to seem jaded by telling their sons. But when a young man brings home the neighborhood stank, his mother will have an attitude toward the female, and the son will have no clue why.

The reality is, many mothers know if your wife, girlfriend, or baby's mama is the neighborhood stank. But most of the time, she doesn't want to say anything, because it would contradict everything she's already told her son about respecting women. As a result, many men have to learn the truth the hard way. There are thousands of men out there who are getting their paychecks garnished (by child support and alimony, etc.) because they chose the wrong woman. And many of these situations could have been avoided if men were taught how to differentiate between a decent woman and a chickenhead. In the next chapter, I will explain exactly how that's done.

What Mothers Teach Their Daughters

As I mentioned before, mothers often teach their sons to place undeserved value on females simply because of their gender. This causes many young men to subconsciously worship and overvalue the vagina. This eventually leads men to place a monetary value on a woman's vagina—in essence, turning men into tricks.

Daughters, on the other hand, are taught the exact opposite. When mothers school their daughters on how to deal with men, the term *respect* isn't even part of their vocabulary. Daughters are told: "You have to use what you got to get what you want," "Don't get with a man who can't get nothing for you," "You better get as much as you can while you can," etc.

Many men have no idea that this is what mothers tell their daughters. But the women who are reading this know exactly what I'm talking about. Girls are taught at a young age that they should use their physical and sexual attributes to get material things from men, and to value a man's occupation over his character. Girls grow up hearing things like, "When you get older you need to marry a doctor or a lawyer." The message this sends to a young girl is that she should offer herself sexually to the highest bidder—in other words, she should become a ho.

To Be a Mack, You Must Understand the Importance of Man

To many, the mackin' game seems extremely far-fetched. The thought of a man having his choice of a number of top-notch women seems incredible to the average square. The thought of a man having total control of not only one woman, but *several* women, seems even more far-fetched. But a lot of rules of the mackin' game are simply based on different Eastern philosophies of dealing with women.

Even today, there are many places in Africa where men live harmoniously with several different wives. In some Arab societies, men still have harems of women and are openly accepted. In many Asian countries, the women are infamous for being submissive to their men. (This is why many American men have Asian-girl fantasies.)

Why is it that in the West, the women control their men, while in the East, the men control their women? What is it that the American hustlers and men of the East know, that the average square man in the West doesn't?

It's simple: True macks understand the importance of a man, and no one understood it as well as the first macks.

The First Macks

The first macks were the ancient Egyptians. Ancient Egyptian men were the first to have game. This translated into having power, wealth, and a number of women. If you look at many of the Egyptian paintings today, you will see pharaohs and kings chillin' with a number of women by their sides.

The Egyptians patterned their lifestyle after the great cats of Africa. It is common knowledge that the ancient Egyptians worshipped cats. One of the most popular structures in Egypt to this day is the Sphinx, a giant stone carving of a pharaoh's head on a lion's body. The Egyptians patterned their relationships after the patriarchal structure of the lion kingdom. The male lion has long been considered the king of the jungle. The male lion is one of the most respected and feared animals in the wild. And what does the male lion do? He chills, for the most part.

The male lion doesn't have to prove his dominance at all times. The male lion sleeps through most of the day, and yet he's the most respected animal in the jungle. The male lion also has a number of female lions that do his work for him. The female lion does all the hunting. The female lion raises the cubs. After the female lion makes a kill, she won't even eat before the male lion has had his fill.

How Your Value as a Man Increases with Time

Throughout history, men have primarily been valued for their game, and women have primarily been valued for their physical attributes. Of course, there are many exceptions to this rule, but the general fact remains that the most popular women throughout history, and even today, such as Cleopatra, Helen of Troy, Marilyn Monroe, and Halle Berry, were and are revered primarily for their physical beauty, while the most popular men throughout history, such as Plato, Imhotep, Socrates, and Malcolm X, have been revered for their knowledge and game. Now, because many women are generally valued based on their physical attributes, their value often decreases as they get older. The exception is the rare female who really takes care of herself.

Since men are valued for their game, their value increases as they get older. It's almost inevitable that they will attain more knowledge as they age. And a man with a higher level of game—which often leads to financial success—is highly desirable to women. The problem is that many young men will jump into a relationship with any low-budget hoodrat who looks their way, because these young men don't realize that their value will eventually increase. A woman at eighteen generally has more value than a man at eighteen. Eighteen-year-old women are more sure of themselves, because at that age they are at the top of the food chain. Everyone is trying to spit at them. Eighteen-year-old women are the most desirable because they are like cars fresh off the lot. They look good. They don't have a lot of miles on them. Eighteen-year-old women have all the things men want: perky breasts, tight booty, no kids (in most cases), and no emotional baggage.

Meanwhile, an eighteen-year-old man sits at the bottom of the food chain. He doesn't really have much of what women want: a career, a car, paper, his own crib. Unless his game is just hella tight, the eighteen-year-old male will have to reduce himself to dating local hoodrats.

As men and women get older, the tables turn. That same eighteen-year-old female will have less value, generally speaking— there *are* exceptions, so no e-mails please, ladies—when she reaches forty. By that time, her body won't be as tight as it was. She will probably have had children. She might have accumulated some emotional baggage. These are all the things men *don't* want.

On the other hand, a man at forty is on top of his game. He has a career. He is more focused. He has a home, a car, and money to spare. In short, he has all the things that women desire. Women always say that men are the sexiest in their forties. If you look at Hollywood, all the top male sex symbols are forty or older. Consider George Clooney, Harrison Ford, Brad Pitt, Mel Gibson, Denzel Washington, or Sean Connery.

As a man, you have to view yourself as being a work of fine art. View yourself as real-estate potential. As we all know, fine art and real estate become more valuable as time progresses.

Value Your Dick

A very important rule that many men in "the life" understand is that a mack must have standards. And a man must value his dick more than he values a coochie. So many square guys today are so glad and grateful that a female (*any* female, at that) will give them some coochie that they are willing to lower their standards.

As a mack, you don't just stick your dick up in any broad. There are guys out there who will literally sleep with *anything*. (These are the Scavengers mentioned in the last chapter.) Now granted, as men, we have all fallen off the wagon every now and then and had sexual relations with a few ducks. But I'm referring to guys who step to below-average women all the time. I'm not talking about the female you banged when you had "Hennessy-vision."

When you keep on stepping to women who are obviously below your standards, you send a subconscious message to yourself that you are not worthy of a quality woman. You're telling yourself that you don't deserve someone better.

As a mack, you must understand that you have two important seeds that you give a woman. One is the seed of "game." This is the verbal knowledge that you plant in her fertile mind. And the operative word is *fertile*.

When you are in a relationship with a woman, she should follow your lead, not the other way around. In order for her to follow you, you must first have your game together (which is what you're doing now by reading this book), and then you must make your thoughts, views, game, and knowledge her views as well. You must plant your ideology in her mind. This way you both will be on the same page.

Your second seed is the biological seed, your sperm cell. Once you grasp the importance of your two seeds and how valuable they are to women, you will have gained full mackdom. The more successful you become and the more game you acquire over the years, the more valuable both of your seeds will be to women.

When a man and woman have sexual relations, who gets the most out of the deal? The man, or the woman? Since we live in a society full of tricks, the man thinks he gets more out of the encounter. But what do men *really* get out of it? The reality is that women have the potential to get more out of it than the man, especially if the man's seeds have accumulated a certain amount of value.

Coochie is just entertainment. It's not a commodity. It's not an asset. It's just a moist, warm hole. You get up in there and entertain yourself for twenty to thirty minutes and that's it. You come back with nothing but the satisfaction of entertainment. But a woman can have sexual relations with a man, acquire his seed, and then live off that seed for the rest of her life. This is especially true for men who are very successful, because their seeds have extra value. You've seen how females will flock to successful ball players or other types of entertainers at clubs, trying to compete with one another to have sexual relations with them. Many women are competing for that one seed. They know that seed is a meal ticket for life.

It's gotten so deep now that many professional sports teams are having seminars for their rookies, hiring people to warn the players about getting caught up. Athletes are now warned to use their own condoms when they go on the road, because there are females who will poke holes in condoms to intentionally try to get pregnant. Athletes are also warned to flush condoms down the toilet after they use them, because females have taken condoms out of trash cans and used the contents to get pregnant.

Obviously, many women are hip to the true value of dick (especially successful dick). Square men, however, have been tricked into believing the opposite. Women know the importance of that seed and that they have a limited time to get it. Once a woman's biological clock starts ticking, if she hasn't gotten that seed yet, she starts "cramming for the test," so to speak. In a recent interview, Halle Berry said that she was going to get pregnant at forty with whatever guy she was with at the time.

As men, we don't have a biological clock, so there isn't much pressure on us to procreate. As a mack, value your seeds and your dick, especially once you have achieved financial stability. Don't rush to give up your seeds, or you could end up paying someone for the rest of your life.

Many people might look at pimp philosophies as misogynistic and disrespectful to women. But understanding your value as a man doesn't mean you have to devalue women. Even though many women won't admit it, they like a man who knows his value. They like a man who won't bow down to them for giving him sex. Many women like the challenge of being with a man who knows his value, and who makes his women earn his attention and devotion.

Know your importance and value as a man. If you want to be treated like a king, you have to act like one.

Top Five Celebrity Men Who Are Known Tricks

1. Charlie Sheen
2. Ben Affleck
3. Drew Carey
4. Kelsey Grammer
5. Hugh Grant

4

HOW TO MACK ON DIFFERENT TYPES OF FEMALES

got an e-mail from a guy recently, which read:

K-Flex,

I'm from an upper-middle-class neighborhood in South Carolina. I've dated a few girls from my area, and for the most part, things went pretty well. I would always be nice and sweet to them, and they seemed to really appreciate that. The problem is this: I moved out of that area, and now I'm going to school in Florida. The females here are more fast-paced and hip, I would say.

I've tried to date a few females down here, but when I try to treat them nice and sweet like I did with the females back home, they seem to lose interest. Not only do they lose interest,

*but it seems the nicer I treat them, the more they lose respect
for me. What's the deal, Flex? Do I need to become an a-hole
just to get some play down here?*
Signed,
"Confused Down South"

His problem is the same problem a lot of players face: He has to
learn how to switch up his game. You must understand that, as a
mack, you simply can't treat every female the same way. You can't
be too thuggish with a suburban female, and you can't be too
sweet to a hoodrat. As a mack, you almost have to be schizo-
phrenic. You have to be a chameleon. You have to be able to change
up your game at the drop of a hat. This will also help you keep females off-guard and unable to figure you out. Women love mysterious men. Once they see that they cannot get a clear handle on
you, they will become even more intrigued.

Identifying the Different Types of Females

In order for your game to be most effective, you must identify and
fully understand the types of females you are stepping to. The true
mack cannot waste valuable time trying to push a square peg into
a circle. Your game has to be suited to the intended target.

Women have often been compared to jewelry, as both are valued on the basis of their beauty, quality, and depth. To help give
you an understanding of the different types of females, I'm going
to show you how they rank, based on the jewelry chart. In addition

to their physical descriptions, I'm going to assess their personalities.

There are five general types of women:

1. Diamond Girls
2. Platinum Honies
3. Gold Hotties
4. Copper Chicks
5. Cubic-Zirconium Broads

In the descriptions below, I give some examples of female celebrities that share the qualities of each type. I have chosen these celebrities not for their level of success, but rather for their backgrounds. Background is often more important in determining a female's type. Some cubic-zirconium–type females become financially successful but continue to have cubic-zirconium ways. I also rate these women on their "beauty shelf life," the time frame in which they remain attractive, based on how well they care for themselves.

Here is an assessment of all five types.

Diamond Girls

Average yearly income: $250,000+
Average weight: 95–130 lbs.
Number of children or abortions before the age of 23: 0
Beauty shelf life: 16–60
Examples of Diamond Girls: Halle Berry, Janet Jackson

General Description

Diamond Girls are the cream of the crop as far as females go; they are the most attractive and most disciplined. Not surprisingly, these females are extremely rare. Many come from very affluent families with upper-echelon backgrounds.

But many females from other backgrounds have worked their way up to diamond status. On a scale of one to ten, these women rate between a nine and a dime. Diamond Girls maintain their good looks for a long period of time because they usually have very disciplined eating habits and workout regimens. These women don't usually engage in excessive drinking, cigarette smoking, or drug use. They are usually very well-educated and surprisingly down-to-earth.

How to Step to a Diamond Girl

A lot of girls are impressed by guys who have achieved status and material success. But not Diamond Girls. These women are not impressed that you have a Benz, because they can afford to drive one, too. Most men think women like this are out of their league. So not surprisingly, not many men step to them. And the guys these women do meet are usually the nerdy guys who are part of their affluent communities of family and friends. She's got plenty of material things, but what's really missing in her life is a guy to have some cool, down-to-earth conversation with. So with Diamond Girls, what you need as a mack is some decent convo. To get with one of these females, your conversation skills have to be trump-tight.

When you step to Diamond Girls, get them to talk about themselves and their backgrounds. Read a few books about geography, because most Diamond Girls have traveled to different places around the world. Being able to discuss some of the places you have been or the places you would like to go is a great way to build a rapport with the Diamond Girl.

Platinum Honies

Average yearly income: $50,000–$150,000
Average weight: 95–140 lbs.
Number of children or abortions before the age of 23: 0
Beauty shelf life: 17–45
Examples of Platinum Honies: Beyonce, Tyra Banks

General Description

Platinum Honies are attractive females who come from upper-middle-class family backgrounds. They come from very stable homes and most grow up with both parents in their lives. As far as looks go, Platinum Honies rate between eight and ten on a scale of one to ten. Many Platinum Honies have accumulated good social skills and self-discipline over the years. They've done this by participating in different extracurricular activities while growing up, such as sports, dance classes, or piano lessons. And because of their self-discipline, many of these women also maintain their good looks well into their forties and sometimes fifties.

Platinum Honies are very easy-going, and also well educated.

Many of these women usually end up in upper-management or supervisory positions at their jobs. They tend to be very responsible and thoughtful.

How to Step to Platinum Honies

Because Platinum Honies are so used to being the boss in their work environment, they often try to bring that bossy mentality into their relationships. As a mack, you have to check that at the door. Like most women, if a Platinum Honey sees that she can boss you around, she will eventually lose respect for you.

When you initially get with a Platinum Honey, she will try to call the shots as far as who calls who first and where you two will go on your first date. Always stand your ground. You have to be very firm with the Platinum Honey. You need to set up the time and place where you two hook up. You need to show her that you are not intimidated by her domineering demeanor. Beneath the surface, Platinum Honies are very sweet and sensitive women who appreciate a man who knows how to be a good leader.

Gold Hotties

Average yearly income: $30,000–$80,000
Average weight: 98–150 lbs.
Number of children or abortions before the age of 23: 0–1 child;
     0–1 abortion
Beauty shelf life: 17–36
Examples of Gold Hotties: J. Lo, Britney Spears, Alicia Keys

General Description

The Gold Hottie usually comes from a lower-middle-class background. The Gold Hottie may or may not have grown up with both parents in the household, but still remains very close with her family. As far as looks go, on a scale of one to ten, most of these females rate between a six and a nine. They are fairly well educated, but unlike the Diamond Girls and the Platinum Honies, who were taught to be self-sufficient, the Gold Hottie is usually encouraged to marry up. They are usually pressured all their lives (subtly and not so subtly) by their families to find a husband by the age of thirty.

Many of these women will go to college and take "decoy classes" (enrolling in an easy class to give the appearance that they are really trying to get degrees) until Prince Charming comes along to save them.

How to Step to Gold Hotties

The Gold Hotties have to be "sweet-macked." You have to be very smooth with your approach. Since the Gold Hottie is used to a close family structure, you have to give the impression, true or not, that you are familial as well. You have to offer the gold female the white-picket-fence fantasy. You have to come across like your main goal is to settle down and raise a Huxtable type of family. You have to be the ultimate Mr. Goody Two-Shoes with the Gold Hottie.

Be sure not to come off too square or nerdy. If you're too gentle, you will turn her off, and if you're too aggressive, you will scare her away. To get the Gold Hottie, you have to find that balance of smoothness. (For the record, when you get a Gold Hottie, you have to keep her mentally disciplined. Many of these women tend to let themselves go after they get married, which is why many of them hit the wall at around thirty-five or thirty-six.)

Copper Chicks

Average yearly income: $12,000–$20,000
Average weight: 100–180 lbs.
Number of children or abortions before the age of 23: 1–2 children;
    0–2 abortions.
Beauty shelf life: 15–28
Examples of Copper Chicks: Mary J. Blige, Eve, Trina

General Description

Copper Chicks are females who grew up in low-income environments. These females are basically victims of circumstance. Even though they were born and raised in the ghetto, Copper Chicks actually *do* try to make an effort to get out of the hood. They use the fact that they grew up in a less than stellar environment as motivation to work hard and become successful in order to have a better life. As far as looks, on a scale of one to ten, most Copper Chicks rate between a four and a strong eight.

Some Copper Chicks may have "cashed out" early and had a kid at a young age. "Cashing out" happens when a female feels like she might not have a strong financial future on her own, so she has a kid in order to guarantee she will at least get the basic necessities out of life: food, medical care, housing from the state, or child-support checks.

Even though many Copper Chicks do try to work hard to create better lives for themselves, there are some Copper Chicks who try to live out their Cinderella fantasies. This fantasy is usually reserved for more attractive Copper Chicks. These females depend solely on their looks to try to attract a Prince Charming (athlete or entertainer) who will rescue them from the hood.

How to Step to Copper Chicks

There are two types of Copper Chicks: the exceptional Copper Chick, and the basic Copper Chick. The exceptional Copper Chick is the very motivated and hardworking one. The basic Copper Chick is the cute girl in the hood who is trying to find Captain Save-a-Ho.

You have to step to the exceptional Copper Chick very boldly. You have to be hip, slick, and fast with your words. This is an inner-city female you're dealing with, so she is used to all types of scrubs stepping to her with lame game. These females have a low tolerance for time-wasting BS. When you step to her, you have to be bold, quick-witted, and able to quickly get your point across.

Now, basic Copper Chicks are a little simpler to step to, because these women have very simple needs. Their desires are basically primitive because they only aspire to get food and shelter, and they are impressed by shiny things, such as gold teeth, rims, jewelry, etc. All you need to do is to pull up in an Escalade with rims holding a bucket of chicken and the basic Copper Chick is all yours.

Cubic-Zirconium Broads

Average yearly income: under $10,000 (including food stamps and
WIC vouchers)
Average weight: 120–300 lbs.
Number of children or abortions before the age of 23: 1–4 children;
1–3 abortions
Beauty shelf life: 14–21
Examples of Cubic-Zirconium Broads: Lil' Kim, Courtney Love

General Description

The Cubic-Zirconium Broad is at the bottom of the barrel when it
comes to females on the dating scene. These are the females you see
on the *Maury Povich* show, trying to figure out who fathered their
children. These are the females who come from a low-income,
ghetto/trailer-park environment, and who are totally comfortable
remaining in that environment. Even if they luck up and make it
out of the hood, they will still carry that ghetto mentality with
them. These women are commonly known as "chickenheads," or in
the white community, "trailer trash."

As far as looks go, on a scale of one to ten these females usually
range from a one to a four. They are described as Cubic-Zirconium
Broads because, like an actual cubic zirconium, many of these females try their best to look like diamonds without fooling anyone.
And just like cubic zirconium, nothing on these females is real.
These women rock fake hair, fake nails, colored contact lenses, and
they wear excessive amounts of makeup.

Because of all the bad food the Cubic-Zirconium Broad eats in her life—government cheese and food with hormones in it, for example—females like this usually develop at a very young age. This is why, when you go to the hood, it's not unusual to see a fourteen-year-old girl who looks like she is twenty-three.

Another way to spot chickenheads is by checking out their navels. Many chickenheads had mothers who didn't know how to properly remove their umbilical cords when they were babies. (You can't use cocoa butter to help remove the umbilical cord.) This causes their navels to protrude or become slightly disfigured as they grow up. Beware.

And because most of these females grow up in homes headed by single mothers with no father figures in sight, Cubic-Zirconium Broads often have "daddy issues." Many of these women will do whatever it takes to get male attention. This is often the basis of the hoochie attire and behavior that chickenheads engage in. Most chickenhead behavior is passed down from generation to generation—from the grandmother to the mother to the daughter.

Chickenheads become sexually active at very young age. They also "cash out" and have babies at a young age, as well. A general rule is "the broker the family, the younger the mother." This is true in impoverished communities all over the world. I've seen it in the United States, South America, the Caribbean, the Pacific islands, the Philippines, etc. If a girl comes from a family that makes less than $10,000 a year, that girl is likely to get pregnant by the age of nineteen. Many of these women also have a number of abortions under their belt. Many of them get abortions only because they aren't sure who their baby's daddy is.

When people have a mentality that has developed in poverty,

their primal instincts take over. The basic primal instincts of any living species are to eat and to procreate; it's self-preservation. This is how chickenheads think. They aren't really concerned with "coming up" in life. They are 100 percent comfortable with getting their basic needs met by others, and nothing more. These women can spend years living in their mama's houses, having babies, getting drunk, smoking weed all day long, and dating every felon in the hood.

How to Step to Cubic-Zirconium Broads

You don't. When you see a Cubic-Zirconium Broad, run for the hills. Remember, as a true mack, you must have standards. You never lower yourself just to get a quick, easy piece of ass, which is the only reason why any man would step to a cubic-zirconium female in the first place.

Guys see that it doesn't take much effort to get one of these females. Chickenheads, surprisingly, have an abundance of men trying to holler at them. This gives these females a false sense of confidence. This is why many chickenheads, as tore-up as they are, try to come across like they are the bomb.

When you kick it with a chickenhead, it sends out a message about you. It says that you are broke. It says that you are desperate. It says that you have low self-esteem. And these same messages that you send to others are internalized in your own mind. So value yourself as a man, and never settle for chickenheads.

Now, some of you guys are in relationships with chickenheads and you don't even know it. Some Cubic-Zirconium Broads try to disguise their true chickenhead persona. And to the untrained eye, they can sometimes come across as normal females. To help you out, I'm going to give you a list of clues. If three or more items on this list apply to a female, she is a bona fide chickenhead.

Twenty Ways to Tell If a Female Might Be a Chickenhead

1. If she is in her twenties, her mother is in her thirties, and her grandmother is in her forties.
2. If she enrolled in school strictly for the student loan money.
3. If she is over the age of thirty and still wearing "baby hair."
4. If she lives in the projects, but has a big-screen TV.
5. If she thinks she looks like Halle Berry just because she's light skinned.
6. If she thinks she looks like Naomi Campbell just because she's dark skinned.
7. If she thinks she looks like J. Lo just because she's Hispanic.
8. If she has had four or more home numbers, cell numbers, or pager numbers disconnected in a three-month time span.
9. If she weighs 93 lbs. and still has a beer gut.
10. Any black girl with blond hair.
11. Any white girl with braids.
12. If she claims she doesn't have a job because she doesn't have transportation or a baby-sitter, but she always seems to miraculously find a babysitter *and* transportation to get to the club every week.
13. If she drinks Sunny Delight.
14. If she has "combination hairstyles" (braids/fingerwave, or Press-n-Curl/feathered, etc.)

15. If she's at the club "crip-walking" in high heels. (I swear I have actually seen this before.)
16. If she doesn't work out at the gym because she doesn't want to sweat out her weave.
17. If she knows how to play spades.
18. If she thinks people who make more than ten dollars an hour are "bougie."
19. If she has to run errands for the day and they all take place at the swap meet.
20. If she puts hot sauce on potato chips.

Other Subcategories of Females to Look Out For

In addition to the five main "precious gem" categories of females, there are a few other types you should be familiar with. Here are a few:

The Bohemian/Hippie Chick

These are the incense-burning, earthy, herbal tea–drinking females who pride themselves on being all-natural and real. These women are well-educated and artistic. The "Boho" female is usually deep into music like India.Arie, Jill Scott, Music Soulchild, Floetry, the Roots, and the whole neo-soul movement.

If you want to get up on one of these type of females, you simply have to show an interest in her creative side. Get her to read you some of her poetry. I've never met a Bohemian/Hippie Chick who didn't write poetry. She will love to be given an opportunity to show off her creativity. Once you get your foot in the door, you are in.

Beware of some of the fake Bohemian/Hippie Chicks. Some Bohos are into the earthy lifestyle because they have a sincere affinity for nature. It's cool to see females who are confident enough in themselves that they don't have to wear a lot of makeup, weaves, and acrylics to be attractive. This should be admired. But there are a lot of Bohemian/Hippie Chicks who get into that lifestyle just to justify being severe weedheads. And true macks don't mess with weedheads.

The Trend Freak

These are the females who try a little too hard to look trendy. A lot of these females are wannabe supermodels, and they try to come across like fashion experts. Many of the Trend Freaks watch music videos all day so that they can emulate the clothing styles they see.

These are the women you see in the club sporting H. Todd boots, a Prada belt, a Louis Vuitt bag, a Burberry hat, and some Chanel glasses. These women are also major attention freaks, as well.

As a mack, you should not take these women too seriously. Despite their over-the-top attire, many of these Trends Freaks are insecure followers. They are often extremely prone to peer pressure, and base their whole existence on what other people might think of them. As a mack, you are 100 percent secure with yourself, and you should look for females who are sure of themselves and can think independently. You don't want to get with a female who is too easily influenced by peer pressure. The worst thing a mack can do is waste time lacing a female with good game, only to have his game salted because the female was too easily influenced by one of her hating homegirls.

Single Mothers

I get tons of e-mails from fellas all over the country asking me whether it's cool to date single mothers. This issue is a real touchy one. There are many things to consider when it comes to dating single mothers. Some of the important factors include:

- **How old was she when she had her first child?**

- **Was she married when she had children?**

- **How many baby-daddies are in the picture?**

If a female had a kid at a very young age (during her teens), this shows signs of irresponsibility. The chances of her "accidentally" getting pregnant again before the age of twenty-seven increase tremendously. And you don't want to be there when she gets "accident-prone."

It's cool to date a single mother who had a kid (or kids) while she was married. This shows that she was at least responsible enough to try to do it the right way. If she has had two or more children by two or more different guys (without being married) before the age of twenty-eight, this is a major red flag. Don't even step to a female like this. She has already made two "mistakes." (These females never own up to the fact that they were most likely *trying* to get pregnant.) And if you get with this type of female, you're just a mistake waiting to happen.

Some single mothers are cool to date because they are more mature and responsible than women without children. They have to take life more seriously, so they really don't have time to BS around and play games. Single mothers like this are the ones who have their own places and get up and work every day to take care of their children. There's nothing wrong with getting with a female like this.

What you shouldn't get with is a female who has a kid while she is laying up in her mama's house. If you come across a female like this, run for the hills. Also, if you meet a female, and all the women in her family have had children at a very young age without being married, she is going to follow suit. The apple never falls too far from the tree.

Now if you're the kind of guy who is specifically looking for a woman with kids because you have a number of kids of your own and you want to put together some kind of ghetto Brady Bunch, well, knock yourself out. Good luck to you. But if you want to play this mackin' game correctly, and you don't want your paychecks to be garnished in the future, then you should seriously take heed to the info I just gave you on dating single mothers.

Older Women

This is another taboo subject in the dating scene. A lot of very young guys send me e-mails asking me whether or not it is cool to date older women. As I mentioned earlier, many younger guys haven't really come into their own yet, so their dating options are often limited.

There are lots of older women who blatantly flirt with younger guys just to get a reaction. These older women do this just so they can be reassured that they still "got it." So for the most part, you shouldn't take their flirting too seriously. Let "Nana" go on about her business.

Now there are some situations where a younger man dates an older woman and it's cool. As long as it *looks* appropriate, there shouldn't really be a problem. As long as the guy is not too young and the female is not too old. In the movie *How Stella Got Her Groove Back,* Taye Diggs and Angela Bassett *looked* appropriate together. Ashton Kutcher and Demi Moore *look* appropriate together.

Now, if Nick Cannon decided to date Della Reese, that wouldn't look appropriate. And if they were an item, people would assume they both had some serious psychological issues. So to all of you who are in your late teens or early twenties, there's nothing wrong with dating an older woman with a youthful, vibrant spirit who has taken good care of herself. But you don't want to get with an old broad who is still trying to be a hoochie. Because there is nothing worse than an elderly chickenhead.

Here is a quick list of **eight ways to tell if you are dating an *old* chickenhead:**

1. If she goes to the club wearing a Troop jacket and leg warmers
2. If she has a gray finger wave
3. If she refers to herself as "a bad mamma-jamma"
4. If she flirts with her pharmacist for free medicine
5. If her kids baby-sit each other
6. If she thinks Lou Rawls is "fine"
7. If she drinks Cold Duck
8. If she is at the club doing the Electric Slide to every song

5

RULES OF THE GAME

I always say, the best form of security is prevention. When you are laced with the proper rules and tools of the game, you tremendously reduce the risk of getting caught up or cut down. Many guys have to learn some of these rules the hard way. Sometimes this takes years of trial and error, and some errors cannot be rectified. By the time some guys learn these rules, it's too late. So here are ten general rules of the game that a mack or potential mack must abide by.

Rule One:
Never talk down on another player.

Women are very perceptive about the things they see men do. When a man who is in the game talks down on another player, the females know what's really going on. Only guys who are insecure have to blatantly throw salt on another player's game.

Now granted, if two players are campaigning to be chosen by the same female, there will always be a bit of mudslinging here and there. Even presidential candidates do this. But if your opponent gets elected, you have to congratulate him, shake his hand, and charge it to the game.

This rule originates from the pimp game. In order to maintain the fraternal camaraderie between the players, many pimps form somewhat of an unspoken bond with one another. (Real true-to-the-game pimps, that is.) They do this so that females can't try to play the pimps against one another, like they do with square guys.

Women play square guys against each other all the time. Throughout history, wars have been started because of females who played square guys against one another. The story of Helen of Troy (as portrayed in the movie *Troy*) is a good example: A war was started because Helen's husband found out that she crept off with another dude in the middle of the night. Likewise, in the movie *Casino,* based on a true story, a group of mafia bosses had Las Vegas on lock. But they lost it all because the guys who were supposed to be in charge started getting sloppy. The wife (played by Sharon Stone) of Robert De Niro's character started having an affair with his best friend (Joe Pesci's character). This created a rift between these two friends that made it easy for law enforcement to infiltrate them. And this caused them to eventually lose the empire they created in Las Vegas.

Similarly, the war between the Crips and the Bloods is rumored to have started when two rival gang members were fighting over a female back in the early seventies. Two square cats can be friends for thirty years, and then let that friendship go straight to hell over a female.

Many cats that are in jail now are in there because of some love triangle. Ironically, you have guys scrappin' with each other over a female, and when they get thrown in jail, the female they were fighting over is out there, kickin' it with the next two fools.

Players in the game don't let it go down like that. If another player's woman steps to a pimp and chooses him, that pimp has to "serve" that player. That means he has to call that player and officially let him know that his woman is now with him. That's a very important part of the code of the game. This will avoid a lot of "he-say, she-say" confusion, and prevents the female from going back and forth between both pimps. Also, many pimps require a female to give up a "choosing fee" when she steps to them, so that the female can't afford to go from pimp to pimp.

Never hate on another player. Show people that you're confident enough to give another player some props. There are only a few true macks out there. And like the old saying goes, it's lonely at the top. There's a lot of room at the top, but it's jam-packed on the bottom. So if you are on top, you really have no reason to hate on those at the bottom.

Rule Two:
Never use sympathy to try to pull females.

As I mentioned before, many men of this generation were raised by single mothers, and they learned how to interact with women from their mothers. As children, whenever these guys wanted something from Mommy, they would whine, pout, cry, or do whatever it took to get her sympathy.

This usually works like a charm, because many mothers are overly sympathetic when it comes to their sons. This is why we have a generation of mama's boys. When guys grow up, they interact the same way they did with their mom as with women they want to date, and they end up getting a rude awakening. The sympathy approach rarely works on women outside your family.

When guys complain to women about how lonely they are or run game about how they lost their jobs, how they just got out of jail, how the white man won't give them a break, or how they are struggling artists trying to make ends meet, it's often a useless hustle. These guys think that these women will hear their sob story and date them out of pity. Usually, however, this just makes these guys look weak.

Mackin' represents strength. A true mack never looks for a "mommy" figure in a woman he's interested in dating. A mack should always appear mentally strong enough to keep himself together. This shows leadership, and women are programmed to look for men with good leadership skills.

Now, there are some women who will fall for the sympathy approach, but they are few and far between. If you roll the dice long enough, you will eventually hit a seven. But you don't step to females relying on luck. A mack steps to a woman using strategy. When you use strategy, you have more control over the outcome.

On the other hand, the sympathy approach can be useful if you come across a female who is looking for a mother/son relationship, and you're trying to get some quick, one-night-stand, smash-and-grab poon-tang. But you can't get into any type of long-term relationship using the sympathy approach. Even if a female does date you out of pity, she will eventually become resentful. Remember, strength goes a long way. Charity doesn't.

Rule Three:
Always let females know that you have options.

One of the greatest tools a mack can have is options. Options, or lack thereof, can make or break a mack. Too many guys allow themselves to be monopolized by females. In many cases, when a female sees that she has a monopoly on you, she will flip the script. She will feel like she can step to you any way she wants to.

This is the case in any situation where there is a monopoly on services. For example, in order to drive, you have to have a state-issued driver's license. The only place where you can get a driver's license is the state-run DMV. The DMV has a monopoly, and the people at the DMV know that you can only come to them for a license. This is why they treat you like crap at the DMV. At any DMV you go to, you will see ridiculously long lines and DMV workers with the worst attitudes, who drag ass when it comes to helping you. What incentive do they have to give you good customer service? You ain't going nowhere. No matter how funky they treat you, you're still going to have to stay there and take it, because you have to.

The same goes for dating. When you're with a female, and she sees that you don't really have the ability to get other females, she will start talking to you any way she wants. And she knows that you'll just sit there and take it. Ultimately, she will lose respect for you. She will nitpick you about everything, degrade you, and eventually she'll kick you to the side.

As a mack, you have to let a female know that she is not doing you a favor by being in the picture. You have to let her know that she can be replaced and your life won't miss a beat without her. You don't have to do this verbally. When you verbally let females know about your options, they can usually see that it is an obvious bluff. Saying things like "I've got other girls who would want me, too," isn't convincing at all. You have to show her with your actions.

When you keep yourself well maintained, and you keep your paper flowing, you automatically get real options. If you generally stay fly, and carry yourself like the top-notch mack you truly are—even you married macks can do this—you will always have females checking for you.

A man with options will keep a female minding her P's and Q's. When a female knows she can easily be replaced, she is less likely to come at you out of pocket. This is another reason why women are determined to get their men to commit to marriage. Women know that once a man is married, there are legal repercussions for him if he cheats. This is why a lot of men complain that their wives let themselves go, or that their personality changed (i.e., she got bitchy) after they got married.

Married women do tend to switch their game up after the wedding, because in their minds they know "they got you." In this legalistic day and age, a lot of guys figure, "it's cheaper to keep her." Always have options when it comes to females. Even though a lot of women won't admit it, they like the thought of winning over a man who is in demand with other ladies. Women are very competitive with one another, and knowing that she snagged you from the pack gratifies a woman's ego. Being sought-after goes a long way in your relationships with women.

Rule Four:
Always be a mystery.

To be a true mack, you must personify exceptional qualities, or at least create the *illusion* that you have exceptional qualities. You have to come across as if you are greater than a mortal man. When you walk into a room, your mere presence should stir up excitement. As a mack, you almost have to come across like a superhero. The way to do this is to create an air of mystery.

Have you ever wondered why superheroes and comic-book characters are so intriguing? It's because they have an air of mystery. Superman, Batman, and Spider-Man all had women sweating them, because they hid their true identities. These characters have become popular and have generated billions of dollars in merchandising and box-office sales, because women are intrigued by them and men live vicariously through them.

When these superheroes present themselves, they only show their strengths. They show up, save the day by displaying their unique strengths, and then they jet. As a Supermack, that's the impression you want to leave with people. When you first meet people, they see that you have a strong, positive attitude. They see that you are a winner. They see that you don't have a complaint or problem in the world, or they at least get the impression that you don't.

People love to be around winners. The only thing people should know about you is that you have a lot of positive energy, and it's cool to be around you. And that's all they need to know. The less they know, the more superhuman you seem. Most guys step to women and reveal way too much about themselves. Many guys meet women, and then start inundating them with every little detail about their lives, occupation, hobbies, and daily routines.

Many guys come across too flossy, and they try too hard to impress females. When you reveal too much about yourself, women get turned off. Revealing every little mundane detail about yourself makes you seem desperate and too eager to be accepted.

Remember, less is more. To maintain the air of a Supermack, you must always keep them guessing. There is a reason why you never see the practical, daily activities of superhero characters in comic books and movies. You never see Batman taking the Batmobile to get a tune-up. How would you feel about Batman if you saw him sitting up in Pep Boys? You wouldn't think he was much of a hero. You have never seen Spider-Man taking his spider-suit to the cleaners. You never see Wonder Woman at the gynecologist's office.

You don't want to picture superheroes doing these types of average, everyday things, for the same reason that women aren't gung-ho about interacting with a guy who is just like everybody else. Women long for adventure, and they want a guy who can give it to them. Many women live vicariously through men who have adventurous and outgoing personalities. Even if you are not adventurous and outgoing, all you have to do is keep your mouth shut, be cool, and let females *project* their desires onto you.

The great Sigmund Freud, father of modern psychoanalysis, once noted that many of his female patients began to fall in love and have strong sexual desires for him over a period of time. This baffled him for a while, but then he discovered that these women were simply projecting the desires they had for their parents onto him.

This is why, as a mack, you have to become a psychiatrist in a sense, and get women to reveal their pasts, hopes, dreams, and desires to you. Remember, mackin' is all about attitude.

Rule Five:
You must let a female choose you.

The world's first "squares" were the prehistoric cavemen. The world's first macks were the Egyptian pharaohs. Cavemen were only advanced enough to use their simple, primal instincts. The pharaohs elevated their minds so they could use language and logical thinking. Cavemen used force to get women. Pharaohs used game.

Cavemen would do things like hide in the bushes, wait for a female to walk by, club her over the head, and then drag her by her hair to a cave where they could take advantage of her sexually. On the other hand, women competed for the opportunity to be with a pharaoh. Like many squares today, cavemen were more intrigued by the challenge of chasing women and conquering them. Just like modern macks, the pharaohs were very selective about the women they wanted on their team. They made women compete to be down. Cavemen liked to conquer. Pharaohs liked cooperation.

As a mack, you must think like a pharaoh, and realize all the assets that you have at your disposal. You have to carry yourself in such a way that females will want to choose you. Too many men think that if they chase women, beg them for dates, call them over and over, or pester them non-stop, they will eventually wear the women down. They think these women will eventually give in and be with them.

To a mack, that's too much energy spent without an appropriate payoff. You can save a lot of time, energy, and money simply by finding a female who likes you. If you have to jump through hoops in order for a female to vibe with you, chances are she really doesn't like you anyway.

As a mack, you have to start "posin' to be chosen." You have to put yourself in a position to be chosen by females. Then you have to be able to read nonverbal language. Some women choose men in subtle ways, and some women choose men in more aggressive ways. Some women might step to you and compliment you on the outfit you are wearing. Some women might choose you by a giving you a glance or a seductive stare. You have to pick up on these little things and react accordingly.

Whenever you catch a female doing some subtle choosing, you can feel her out by stepping to her on a courteous level. Throw a simple "Hello, how ya doin'?" at her. Monitor her reaction. If it's warm and receptive, this is her way of choosing. Then you can proceed with more game.

Rule Six:
Put your dick in your pocket.

This rule is an extension of Rule Five. "Put your dick in your pocket," is an old pimp expression, and it has two meanings. When a pimp would encounter a new female, instead of stepping to her with "his dick in his hand," wanting to get sex from the woman like the average trick or square, the pimp would take his dick out of his hand and put it in his pocket, so to speak. With his dick out of the way, he could then pimp at the female accordingly.

The other meaning of this expression is that the only way a female could get sex from a true pimp was if she took care of his pockets (by putting money in there) first. This goes back to valuing yourself as a man.

Once you put yourself in a position to be chosen by a female, you then have to get her to do the chasing. And once you get her chasing, you must continue to make her chase. You do this by being somewhat unattainable. This is challenging for females. And whether they will admit it or not, women like a good challenge in a man.

Most men will immediately put all their cards on the table and roll out the red carpet for females as soon as they meet them. They do this in the hope of getting sex from these women right away. As a mack, you have to trump the pussy card. You have to show a female that she has to bring more to the table than just sexual gratification. You have to reverse the game and have her rolling out the red carpet, jumping through hoops so she can receive sexual and psychological gratification from you. The only way to do this is by keeping your dick in your pocket so it won't get in the way of your game. (More on this later.)

Rule Seven:
Never become financially dependent on a female.

As I mentioned before, many guys today grow up in single-mother homes. Many guys (especially black men) grow up in families where there are nothing but dominant women telling them what to do. When these men become adults, they subconsciously look for that same dynamic in their relationships with women.

Too many guys today are dependent on females for shelter, transportation, food, and all the other basic necessities of life. As a mack, you should never put yourself in this position. Whenever you get into a mother/child relationship with a female, you always put yourself at a disadvantage in the long run. You might think you're living easy because someone else is paying the bills. But the situation can go south when you least expect it. And it usually does.

Many women who get into these mother/child relationships grew up in single-mother homes, as well. These women grew up seeing their mothers run things—in many cases, there wasn't a man who hung around for any long period of time—so these women erroneously assume that women are the dominant ones in relationships. So they subconsciously look for needy men who can be easily controlled.

Contrary to popular belief, women like this are terrified of strong men. They never knew strong male figures growing up, and they realize that a strong man cannot be easily controlled. Since they grew up seeing men going in and out of their mothers' lives, they figure the best way to keep a man around is to find a man who needs and depends on them.

Women like this are perpetually unsatisfied. The catch-22 is that even though they specifically look for men they can dominate, once they find men who will follow them and jump when they say jump, they will eventually lose respect for them.

Women like this will offer you the keys to their crib, the keys to their car, the whole nine. But don't ever fall for the bait. Once a female sees that you're totally dependent on her, she will flip the script on you 100 percent of the time. As a mack, you have to be the boss. Most male bosses are fair and just, and they will only "fire" a female if she deserves it. But a female boss will often fire you simply because she can.

Rule Eight:
Never spend more than $50 on a first date.

Many guys think being flossy and flashy and spending a lot of money on a female when they first meet is going to impress her. But in many cases, the opposite occurs. As I said before, when you try too hard to impress females right after you meet them, you look insecure.

As a mack, you have to come out of your mouth with game before you come out of your pocket with change. It doesn't matter how much money you have in your bank account—you can have $100 or you can have $1 million. Never spend more than $50 on a first date. The first impression is always the lasting one. The way you start off with a female is the way you're going to end up with a female. If you start off trickin', she's going to expect you to keep on trickin'. And if you start off providing good convo, and she is really feeling you, she will expect good game from you from that point on.

You don't spend more than $50 on a first date, because first, you don't want to make too much of the blind investment on someone you really don't know. The female could be cool, or she could be a psycho. You don't know yet. Second, the message you want to send to the female is: "I don't know if I want you on my team yet." You have to subtly let females know that you aren't the kind of guy that has to try to impress people. By spending less than $50 on a first date, you show that you don't have to spend a lot of money to get females' attention and affection.

Now, after you get to know the female, it's cool to spend a little more paper on a date. You do this only if you know that the female will reciprocate. Why spend money on a female who won't spend money on you? If you two are down to spend paper on each other, then you can increase the $50 limit. But on a first date, always keep it under $50. Ideally, you would just spend $20. The true mack has a $50 curve. Anything over $50 on a first date is trickin'.

If the female really likes you, it won't matter to her how much money you spend or where you take her. Just being in your presence is cool enough for her. But when you meet a female who insists (and I mean adamantly insists) that you two go out or that you take her to an expensive restaurant, etc., this female is really not into you. It's even possible that she has a man already, and by insisting that you take her out on a date (and not coming over to your crib) she can feel relieved of any guilt or wrongdoing. In her mind, this doesn't look like any form of infidelity, because "it's just an innocent dinner date." Also, she might just be an undercover chickenhead who is trying to get a free meal. If you encounter a female who demands that you take her to Red Lobster (high-class dining to a chickenhead) you should send her right back to the swap meet where you got her.

When you get with a female, either she likes you, or she doesn't. It doesn't matter how much money you spend. If a female is really feeling you, you can take her somewhere free, and you two will still have a good vibe. You can take her to the park. You can take her to a museum. Many museums are free. If you live in a coastal area, you can take her to the beach. If she wants a red lobster, let her catch one from the ocean herself.

Rule Nine:
Always assume that women under the age of twenty-seven have significant others.

If you meet a fairly attractive female under the age of twenty-seven, you should always assume that she is already in a "situation." Of course, there are exceptions to this rule, but it generally holds true. Females under the age of twenty-seven are either already dating somebody, or having sexual relations with somebody.

Men and women treat relationships like jobs. When a man

quits a job or gets laid off, he wants to stay unemployed for while. He wants to just kick back and chill for a minute before he gets back into the job market. Women like to have another job lined up before they quit the first job. They like to transition from job to job without any breaks in between.

This is how women deal with relationships. Women have a primal need for security. So, many women will have some kind of backup brotha somewhere in the cut. For some reason, men buy into the fable that decent- (and even some not-so-decent-) looking women are just locked up in the house like hermits, not interacting with any other men.

Just like men, women have booty calls, too. The man a female sleeps with most often is her significant other, and it's almost inevitable that women will have some type of emotional attachment with a man she has sex with on a regular basis. Many women who are twenty-eight or older have done the "job-to-job" thing. They understand the consequences of getting into too many relationships too soon. So they are more inclined to take a decent amount of time off from relationships and booty calls, so they can get their minds together. (But there are many women well over the age of twenty-eight who still do the "job-to-job" form of dating, as well.)

When you first meet a female who is under the age of twenty-seven, don't get jealous or upset when you see guys calling her cell phone or her crib. This has nothing to do with you or how tight your game is. These are just her backup cats. Most females like this have them. The only thing you can do is be as mackish as you can be, and let her fully choose, so she can make that transition from her "minimum-wage job" to your "mack-status entry-level position."

Rule Ten:
Never trust a woman who doesn't perform oral sex on you.

This isn't to say that you should trust every woman who *does* perform oral sex on you. But when a woman you are dating refuses to do it, she is sending you a message. Performing oral sex on a man is a woman's ultimate act of submission. She is deferring her own sexual gratification to give him sexual pleasure. The majority of women out there (even those who seem frigid, or come across as being Ms. Goody Two-Shoes) have either performed or are at least willing to perform oral sex.

When a woman you are dating refuses to do so, she is telling you that she is not down for you 100 percent. Either you aren't "the one" for her and she is just with you until something better comes along, or she has someone else who she saves her "special treat" for.

You should never fully trust a female who isn't 100 percent down for you. If you're one of those guys who think that your girl isn't going down on you because "she's not that type of girl" or because she told you she has strong religious beliefs, I want you to close this book, put it down, and go pick up a brochure for Jerry's Kids. You gots to be retarded if you still fall for that old-school game.

Top Five Colognes for True Macks

1. Curve (You wear this when you are in full-fledged mack mode.)

2. Le Male (You wear this when you want to get women in a sexual mood.)
3. Cool Water (You wear this when you are feeling real pimp-ish.)
4. Eternity for Men (This is a nice fragrance to wear during business meetings.)
5. Issey Mayaky (This is a nice first-date fragrance.)

Top Five Colognes a True Mack Wouldn't Be Caught Dead Wearing

1. Brut
2. Old Spice
3. Hi Karate
4. Stetson
5. Preferred Stock

6

HOW TO STEP TO FEMALES IN DIFFERENT SETTINGS

The most intense moment in a mack's career is the moment just before he first approaches a female. It's the same intense feeling that a football player gets minutes before the big game, the same rush a skier gets before plunging down a steep slope, the same surge of adrenaline that a hip-hop artist achieves seconds before stepping on stage, and the same way a boxer feels right before he gets into the ring. Your thoughts and your attitude in those few moments will either make or break your game.

Unfortunately, when it comes to stepping to females, too many guys are defeated by negative thoughts. So before you jump into the ring and start trying to interact with females, you first must find the correct state of mind. This starts with overcoming fear.

Men's Biggest Dating Fear

When it comes to dating, the greatest fear men have is of getting dissed. This debilitating anxiety is the main obstacle standing between a man and his inner mack. This fear is understandable. No man wants to get dissed by a female. Getting dissed is a bitch. It messes with your ego. It chips away at your confidence. It makes you feel insecure. So many guys do everything they can to avoid getting dissed that they end up sacrificing interaction with women entirely.

But these fears are often exaggerated. Many guys let themselves imagine too many "What if?" scenarios. "What if she is out of my league?" "What if she doesn't want me?" "What if she thinks I'm too short?" "What if she thinks I'm too fat?" "What if she thinks I'm too old?" "What if she thinks I'm too broke?"

So, many guys never stop and think, "What if she *is* down?", "What if she *is* feeling my convo?", or "What if she *does* want to hook up?" The likelihood of you getting dissed is extremely minimal if your convo is in order and you play the game correctly.

Getting "Elected" by Females

Stepping to females is just like trying to get elected into a political office. You're running a campaign until you get elected. As a mack, you have to overcome obstacles on the campaign trail. And the biggest obstacles are the ones in your own mind.

You have to realize that no matter what shortcomings you

think you have, you should still focus on your positive attributes. There are many guys out there who clearly have shortcomings, but still get the top-notch females out. To defeat your insecurities, you have to recognize them. The four insecurities men most commonly have are:

1. Their height ("I'm too short")
2. Their weight ("I'm too fat")
3. Their age ("I'm too old")
4. Their financial status ("I'm too broke")

As a mack, you should never let any of these four obstacles keep you from getting the dimes and top-notch females out there. Other men have overcome these obstacles, and so can you. All you need to do is tighten your game up.

If you think you're too short, look at Janet Jackson, one of the finest sistas in the game. Who is she down with now? Lil'-bitty-ass Jermaine Dupree. Some of you might say, "Well, he may be short, but he has Janet because he has money." Well Janet has long money. Plus, her family has paper, too. So Jermaine's paper has no influence on her. You just have to tighten up your game to get a sista like Janet. Jermaine has definitely tapped into his mack within.

If you think you're too overweight to get females, look at brothers like soul singer Gerald Levert. Gerald jumps on stage, belly and all, and women go crazy over this cat. And the late, great Biggie Smalls (R.I.P.), who was an infamously overweight brotha, had women literally fighting over him. Again, you just have to tighten up your game. Biggie was also tapped into his mack within.

If you think you're too old, just go back to chapter three, where

I explained how a man's value increases as he gets older. And peep out old-school players like Warren Beatty and Sean Connery. These cats are way up in age and they are still considered sex symbols. I'll say it again: You just have to tighten up your game.

If you think you're too broke to get seemingly unattainable females, look at Britney Spears. She married two different guys who couldn't rub two nickels together. Once again, you just have to tighten up your game.

If you think your looks are not good enough to get top-notch females, remember Julia Roberts' marriage to Lyle Lovett. She was one of the most attractive actresses in Hollywood at the top of her career when she married musician Lyle Lovett. Lyle looks like an elderly gerbil with a perm. But he was still able to pull Julia Roberts. You have to tighten up your game, just like he did.

All these examples prove that no matter how fly you look, no matter how tall you are, no matter how much money you make, you will eventually get elected—if your game is tight enough, you're comfortable enough with yourself, and you campaign in the right places. That's what this chapter is about.

A Mack Must Use Tact

To be a good mack, you have to be tactful. You can't step to every female the same way. You have to tailor your game to the immediate surroundings. In some situations you have to be a little bolder than usual. In other situations you have to be a little smoother than usual. For example, if you are stepping to a female in a place where she is likely to be in a hurry, it's actually possible to be too smooth with your game. You might have to put your game in third gear and get to the point with the female before she's gone.

Similarly, if you're in somewhat of a laid-back setting, you can be too bold with a female. You can't step to a female at church and say, "Take my number down and holler at a pimp." That would be inappropriate and throw the whole vibe off. This is why you need to understand what level of game to use where.

A Mack's Game Is Like a Ferrari

To understand the different levels of game, look at your mackin' skills like you would a Ferrari, and adjust your speed accordingly. You can't speed in a residential district, and you can't go too slow on the freeway. If your game is too slow for a fast-paced female, she will lose interest. And if your game is too fast for a small-town girl, you will talk over her head and she won't see where you're coming from.

Here are the four "gears" of game you should use when putting the mack down.

First Gear

This is when you step to a female on a courtesy level, giving the appearance that you are not even mackin' at all. This level of the game comes across as harmless and unthreatening. This gear of game is used to monitor the female's vibe. If you can't get an accurate reading on a female, you should stay in first gear. If the vibe is good and receptive, then you should switch to second gear.

Second Gear

This is when you get a positive vibe from a female and you are letting her know, in a subtle way, that you might be interested in taking the interaction to another level. Being in second gear keeps a woman guessing whether or not you really want to holler at her. When you are in second gear, you might flirt with the female or give her compliments on her shoes or jewelry. For the record, you should never step to females with compliments on their physical beauty. If makes you come across as a kiss-ass.

Never step to women saying things like, "I would do anything to be with a woman of your stature." You might as well pull out your wallet and write BIG-ASS TRICK on your forehead, because that's how she'll see you.

When you are in second gear, don't show blatant interest or a strong desire for the female you just met. You must give her the impression that you are still waiting on her to give you a reason to want to take it to the next level.

Third Gear

Putting your game in third gear is when you are ready to express interest in further contact. You see that she is feeling you. She sees that you are feeling her. This is when you exchange numbers or e-mail addresses and arrange to see her again in the near future.

If for any reason you have misread her vibe, and she says something like, "Well I can't give out my number because I have a man," you must put your mackin' gear in reverse, and put it back into first gear. Be sure to pace yourself when you are mackin' to a female. You don't want to shift gears too fast.

Fourth Gear

Your game is in fourth gear when you're vibing with a female so well, you can not only set up future dates with her, but get her to come to your crib or to the "mo-mo" with you, right then and there. Fourth gear is when your game is so tight, you get elected on the spot.

Tailoring Your Game to Different Settings

In my book *The Art of Mackin'*, I dedicated an entire chapter to meeting women in clubs. I used clubs as a forum to meet women, because this is where a mack can easily accomplish his goals.

Over the years, however, I've received tons of e-mails from guys who don't usually go to clubs. In some cases, they're too young to get in clubs, or the clubs in their cities are just wack. These readers have asked me how to meet females in other kinds of spots. I have listed some below, and explained the best "gear" to use when getting your game on in each location.

The Gym

Let's face it: many gyms are pickup spots, especially the ones in L.A. But when you step to females at the gym, you have to put your game in first gear and let it coast for a while. You don't have to be in much of a rush with your game, because people usually take their time and spend at least an hour or two at the gym, anyway. So you can let the mackin' marinate. When you step to females at the gym, you should stay in first gear and come at the female on a courtesy level.

If you step to a female at the gym, make sure she looks like she's been going to the gym for a while. As a mack, if you're at the gym putting the mack down, at least be playa enough to get a top-notch female who is in shape. Don't punk out and try to spit at the pudgy chick that just joined the gym. That's a major no-no. These females already feel very insecure and self-conscious. No matter how tight your game is, the only thing on her mind is "I hope he doesn't notice my big belly," or "I hope he doesn't notice my fat ankles," or "I hope he doesn't notice my jiggly thighs."

When you step to a physically fit female at the gym, you have to tailor your game to the setting. Ask about her workout regimen. Ask her about her nutritional habits. Ask her about her ab techniques. When you step to her, you have to get her to lower her defenses by putting yourself in the position of pretending to need advice. Ask for her advice on a workout routine. People who have worked hard at something that they are proud of (like a female has worked on her body) take great pride in explaining and even bragging about it. You have to use this to your advantage. If you see a female at the gym that you are feeling, simply step over to her and say something like, "I was checking out your arms, and they look well toned. Which machine do you normally use to get your arms like that?"

Now, a comment like this accomplishes two things: 1) It eliminates the fear and possibility of being rejected, because you can't reject courtesy and 2) It gives you an opportunity to monitor the female's vibe and attitude, which lets you know if it's cool to shift your game into second gear.

The Mall

When mackin' to females at the mall, you should once again put yourself in the position of needing assistance from the female. In this scenario, you may have to speed your game up just a taste (but not too fast) because you never know if a female is there to do some window-shopping, or if she's there to quickly pick up a specific item.

At the mall, you have to start off in first gear, and then you have to switch into second and third gear within two to three minutes. The best way to step to females at the mall is using the "I need your opinion" approach. This is the best way to break the ice, keep her defenses down, and get a feeling for her overall demeanor.

Go to the cosmetics counter in a department store and try spraying two or three different colognes on some samples strips, and approach your target on the courtesy level. Say to her, "Excuse me, I need to get a female's opinion on something . . ."—saying this shows you don't have any threatening intentions—". . . I'm trying to decide which new cologne I should get, and I wanted to know which one smells the best to you."

After she responds, you have to pick up on the receptiveness of her vibe toward you. If she is somewhat intelligent, and she is into cats that have decent convo, she should be a little more receptive to you.

If she gives you her opinion but seems like she may be in a rush, don't sweat it. No harm, no foul. Charge it to the game and keep on campaigning. If you get a positive vibe from her, you should then shift from first gear to second gear. After she gives her opinion on which cologne she likes, you then switch the convo to her: "So, who are you here with?" or "What are you picking up here at the mall?" or "How far do you live from here?"

If you are in the main part of the mall, you can use the same approach to break the ice. If you see a female who might be qualified for your game, step to her and say, "Excuse me, you look like you have good fashion sense." This is a very effective statement because females tend to believe they have exquisite fashion sense, and they will feel proud that someone is acknowledging it. Then say, "I'm going to a formal event, and I need to find some upscale gear. I'm not sure which stores I should check out. You look like you would know where there is a high-end fashion store here in this mall."

This icebreaker is very effective. If she says she doesn't know where the upscale clothing stores are in the mall, she is basically admitting that she doesn't have the fashion sense that you think she has. Most females really wouldn't want to come across like that, and therefore they won't mind giving you advice on where to find a high-class fashion spot.

After she gives you her opinion, you again switch to second gear with your game. Once her defenses are down, get to know her name, age, where she lives, etc. And if that flows well, switch to third gear, give her your number (or suggest that you two exchange numbers), and tell her to give you a holla.

Driving Down the Street

When you're driving down the street, and you see a fly honey going about her way or standing at a bus stop, you have to quickly switch your game from first to second to third gear if you want to spit at her.

Now, it's imperative that you start off on a courtesy level with a female who is just walking down the street, because her apprehensions about a stranger approaching her are probably strong. Generally, when women (and especially attractive ones) are walking down the street, they are subjected to all types of catcalls and lame remarks from guys who pass by. As a result, they may feel vulnerable. If you just drive up to a female and say, "Hey, what's your name?" she probably won't even bother to respond (unless she's a hoodrat). As a mack, you have to quickly lower her defenses while you break the ice.

Here is an excellent technique to use when trying to meet females on the street—this usually works like a charm. It's called the "I need directions" technique. What you do is find a piece of paper in your car, and you pretend that there are directions on it. Pull up to the female target, making sure she sees your piece of paper with the "directions" on it, and you say, "Excuse me, how do I get to Third Street (or whatever a well-known street in your city is) from here?"

Make sure that it's not a street that is too obvious to find from your location. After she gives you the directions, and lets her defenses down, you quickly go from first to second gear. Ask her something like, "So, where are you on your way to?" or "You must live around here?" or "What's your name?" Then switch your game to third gear, and suggest that you two exchange numbers so you can converse later on.

This same gear-shifting approach can work anywhere. Just remember to make your initial approach appropriate to the setting.

If you are at a grocery store, and you see a honey, step to her as if you need some advice on how to make lasagna. If you are on the subway and you see a nice little breezy, ask her which train to take to get to a certain part of town. If you see a female at church that you want to step to, ask her if she knows when the new Kirk Franklin CD is coming out.

A mack's biggest obstacle is the initial approach—the ice-breaker. Once you get your foot in the door with these simple examples I've given, it's smooth sailing from there on out.

Tips on Mackin' at the Club

In most settings, the highest level of game the average guy will reach is third gear. But the nightclub is the perfect place to take your game from first to fourth gear in a short period of time. When guys go to clubs, they are trying to achieve one goal: pull a female out of the club, and convince to her leave with them that night. Some guys will settle for a phone number, or a few dances. But the typical goal for a man frequenting a club is to reach the fourth gear of mackin'.

In order to do this, you simply have to find a female at the club who is on the same page as you are. But this simple process is usually thwarted, because men get sidetracked by all the decoys and obstacles in the club. Many guys waste too much valuable mackin' time with the wrong females who have other agendas. In the process, they end up missing out on the "down-ass" females who are qualified to receive good game.

Here are a few of the types of females at the club that you

should become familiar with. When you spot these females, you should quickly avoid them so you will still have time to find a female who is more compatible with your true mack energy. These females are:

1. The Bar Wench
2. The Attention Freaks
3. The Stella
4. The First-of-the-Month Females
5. The Liquor Strippers
6. The Broke Divas

The Bar Wench

The Bar Wench is the female who hangs out by the bar all night and flirts with guys until they buy her drinks. You have to stay on your toes when you run across this type of female. She will give you the impression that she's yours, but in reality, she just wants you to get her a double shot of Hennessy. Then it's on to the next sucker. You can usually peep out a Bar Wench's game because she is a little too touchy-feely and seems to laugh a little too hard at your jokes. She puts on a big charade just to make you buy her a drink.

It's not simply about getting buzzed. This is a little psychological game Bar Wenches play with themselves. In their minds, their desirability is based on the number of guys they can persuade to buy them drinks. As a mack, you don't have time to waste on a Bar Wench who's just trying to get her drink on. When a female like this starts hinting for you to wet her whistle, just excuse yourself and keep it moving.

The Attention Freaks

There are generally two types of hos: money hos and attention hos, also known as Attention Freaks. These are the women who go to clubs and act like hos, carry themselves like hos, and dress like hos, but are seeking attention, not money.

As a mack, don't waste time bothering with Attention Freaks. Their only goal is to dress provocatively (i.e., stank) and come across as being overly sexual party girls so that guys fawn over them. These women are desperate for attention, and they will do anything to make sure they get it.

Attention Freaks usually run in packs of four or five. When you see a group of scantily dressed females that are loud, tipsy, and dancing in a circle with one another, you better go the other way. True macks aren't in the business of pumping up the egos of Attention Freaks.

The Stella

This is an extension of a type of female I described in chapter four. The label derives from the movie *How Stella Got Her Groove Back*. These are the females who are a little long in the tooth but still go out to the clubs to see if they still "got it."

Many of these women have the same agenda as the Attention Freaks. Stellas are insecure about getting older, so they dress all hoochie and go to the clubs and flirt with any and every guy who looks their way. They are trying to get any form of attention from men they can find. When you run into a Stella, just do an about-face and keep on moving.

The First-of-the-Month Females

These are the chickenhead females that normally frequent the clubs on the first and fifteenth of the month. As a matter of fact, you should try to avoid going out to clubs around the first of the month altogether. This is when hoodrats and chickenheads get their county checks. Once these females get their checks, they run to the swap meet to get some new gear and flock to the club. These types of girls can't afford to go to the club any other time of the month. But after they receive those welfare checks, they can afford to get their hair done and hire a baby-sitter.

As a mack, you don't even want to be in that environment. If you are out fishing and you're trying to hook the "big catch," you don't want to do it in a lake full of tadpoles. You don't want to try fishing for bass during guppy season. You don't want to have to keep throwing back fish you don't want. Make sure your waters are clear of the small fish before you go out mackin'.

The Liquor Strippers

These females are an extension of the Bar Wench. The only difference is that the Liquor Strippers work a little harder for their drinks than the Bar Wench does. The Liquor Stripper is the kind of female who takes a guy on the dance floor, grinds all over him, backs her ass up on him, and basically gives him a lap dance as if she's working at a strip club. After she performs her impromptu stripper act on the dance floor, she tries to work the guy over to the bar so she can get him to buy her a drink.

Whenever you are at the club and you have a female dancing up on you a little too stank, be sure to see what her reaction is after the song is over. If she is down to go off in the cut, so you two can further converse, that's cool. But if she starts talking about how thirsty she is, tell her "thanks for the dance," and keep on campaigning.

The Broke Divas

These are the females who go to the club dressed in the latest trendy fashions and pretend that they are much classier than all the other women in the club. These women don't go to clubs to interact with the fellas, because they like to pretend that the guys in the clubs are beneath them. Despite the snooty persona they like to put on, these women live in the same housing projects as all the other chickenheads. Broke Divas like to front like they have it going on, but in reality they don't have a pot to piss in or a window to throw it out of.

Most people (men or women) who really have paper tend to be more low-key. The brokest people are usually the flossiest people. So when you're at the club and you see a wannabe-high-class female walking around in Gucci and Prada gear, don't think you are somehow beneath her. She probably boosted that new Gucci and Prada from the mall earlier that day. Females who really have it going on are usually down-to-earth. And that is what you should be looking for.

Now I know that some of these labels might seem kind of harsh, but in the mackin' game, you have to have a take-no-prisoners attitude. There are guys who literally waste years of their lives dealing with the types of females I have been describing. These men live in frustration, not knowing that the grass is definitely greener on the other side. All these guys have to do is respect the game and soak it in. And when they go out to the clubs, their chances of getting their game into fourth gear will increase tremendously.

A Mack Must Mingle

A lot of men who go to clubs tend to just stand around or post up by the wall. It's cool to post up periodically, but too many guys play the wallflower role all night. And this isn't going to cut it.

See, a mack must mingle. You have to keep it moving. A mack's game is like water. He has to let it flow throughout the club. You can't stand in one place and let your game sit like a puddle, hoping that a female might walk by and step in it. You have to work the room and douse females with little droplets of your game. You do this by stepping to a number of females on the courtesy level.

Just step to females with a quick, simple, "How are you tonight?", "Are you having a good time so far?", "Cool, I'll talk to you in a minute." Using that simple ten-second exchange is like sprinkling the females with a little water of your game. It also accomplishes other things. It gives you a chance to read the female's vibe and helps tell the female whether you are really interested in her. It shows that you are confident enough to step to a female without saying or doing anything that will put mildew on your game. Most importantly, it eliminates the possibility of rejection.

Once you've planted the seed in the minds of a number of your potential recruits, it's now time to add more water so those seeds will grow into trees. If you have gotten a good vibe from one of the females you stepped to on a courtesy level, you go back to her and put your game into third or possibly fourth gear.

It's important to note that a mack must never ask a female if she will do something. A mack must always *instruct* the female to do something. You don't ask a female if she would like to dance. You don't ask a female for her number. You give her instructions on what you want her to do. If you want her to dance with you, you step to her, take her hand and say, "Come on, we're going to dance." If you want a female's number, you tell her, "Look, let's exchange numbers, because we need to talk about some things." This shows that you are confident enough to take charge. Many women, no matter how independent they claim to be, are secretly turned on by this.

This is the mentality you must have when you're out mingling at the clubs. When you're trying to get elected by females, you have to go out there and shake hands and kiss babies, so to speak. It's a must that you mingle and interact with the people whom you want to put you in "office."

Places Where You Shouldn't Try to Mack to Females

Even though a mack should be able to put his bid in at any given moment, there are a few places where you should avoid, or at least be cautious of, putting your mack down. Unless you have an immediate fourth-gear vibe from the females in these locations, I would suggest that you avoid them all together. These places are:

Your Job

The work environment is one of the worst places to try to spit game at females. If you don't plan on being at that job for too long, or if it's just a temp assignment, that's cool. Mack on. But if it's a job with benefits and income that you absolutely depend on, don't do it. It's a bad idea to get with a female at work. Let's say you do date or get into a relationship with a coworker, and it doesn't work out. You still have to see this person, and in many cases, interact with this person every day. The awkwardness will make the work environment uncomfortable.

The best thing to do with females at your job is to use them as matchmakers. Just be cool and cordial with them, and have them hook you up with their friends. And make sure those friends don't work for the same company as you, either.

Strip Clubs

There are many guys who frequent strip clubs, harboring the notion that they are going to possibly luck into some free ass. In reality, the odds of that happening are slim to none. Your chances of taking a female home with you (for free) are much better at a square club than a strip club.

The females at strip clubs are there to hustle. Point-blank. They are not your friends. They only want to interact with guys who are paying them, but true macks don't pay for companionship. Girls at strip clubs only want to interact with tricks or pimps. Unless you have a foot in the pimp game, you shouldn't go to strip joints thinking you are going to get some free ass. Strippers are used to guys trying to bargain and negotiate for sexual favors from them on a nightly basis. Over time, these women build up a certain level of contempt for guys who try to get sex from them.

If you do want to get with a stripper, catch her outside of her work environment. Catch strippers when they are out at square clubs. (More on how to spot undercover strippers and working girls later.)

Females in an Employee/Customer Environment

Not only is it a bad idea to try and holla at strippers while they are at work, you should also be very cautious when you're trying to talk to *any* female while she is at work. Some females work in customer service positions where they *have* to be nice to people. And some guys take this the wrong way.

I believe if you play the mackin' game, you have to play it fair. The mackin' game is about free will. You should always put yourself in a position where if the female is feeling your game, cool, she can sign up. If the female is not feeling your game, cool, she can go on her way. But it's not fair to mack hard to a female who is working the cash register at the grocery store or working at a department store and doesn't have the option to walk away if she is not feeling your game.

There are a lot of guys who will spit some lame game to a female who is working the cash register at a department store. The female is standing there still smiling, grinning, and being friendly, and so the guys mistake this as their game being on-point. In reality, the female has to be friendly and courteous to every customer that comes in the store, no matter what. This makes it very difficult to get an accurate reading on the woman's true feelings. So play the game fair. There are plenty of other females to mack on out there.

Beauty Salons

Women just aren't looking their best when they are at the hairdresser. Women don't even want to be seen while getting their hair done, let alone macked on. This goes for females in nail shops, too. They don't want men seeing them when their feet look like hooves.

Trying to spit at a female who is in the process of getting her hair or nails done is just wasting time. She isn't going to be focused on the quality and splendor of your game. She's going to focus on what you think of her looking the way she does at that moment. What female is in the mood to exchange numbers with a playa when she has half a weave hangin' off her head? If you're going to mack to a female at a beauty salon, at least wait until she gets out from under the dryer before you put your bid in.

Top Five Old-School Joints a True Mack Would Burn onto a CD

1. "Freddy's Dead" by Curtis Mayfield
2. "Between the Sheets" by the Isley Brothers
3. "The Theme from *Shaft*" by Isaac Hayes
4. "Cool" by the Time
5. "Give It to Me" by Rick James

Top Five Old-School Songs a Simp Would Burn onto a CD

1. "Believe" by Cher
2. "Soon as I Get Home (I'll pay your rent, I'll buy your clothes)" by Babyface
3. "Treat Her Like a Lady" by the Temptations
4. "One Last Cry" by Brian McKnight
5. "Wake Me up Before You Go-Go" by Wham

7

MACKIN' MUSTS AND MUST-NOTS

A true mack can't afford to make mistakes in the game. There are many situations where one mistake can prove devastating. There are only two ways to learn the mackin' game: the right way, and the wrong way.

The wrong way is by trial and error. Granted, there are some times in your life where you need to make mistakes so you can learn from them. But there are guys out there who insist on making the same mistakes over and over again, and are surprised when they never get the results they want. For a man, getting into the wrong dating situation with the wrong female can completely alter your life. Just ask all the guys out there who pay alimony, child support, palimony, or money for sexual harassment lawsuits.

The right way to learn the game is by immediately learning from your mistakes and peeping the game of someone who is seasoned and more experienced in the game. You've already made that step by reading this book. This is how I learned the game. If I was uncertain about something, I would put my ego to the side and seek out advice from some of the veterans in the game. If I made a mistake, I made damn sure not to ever make that mistake again.

Now I'm going to help you try to avoid some of the same mistakes that so many potential macks have made in the past. I've compiled a list of seven main mistakes (or "must-nots") that guys make, and I have also included strategies ("musts") to help prevent those mistakes.

1) A mack must accept when something isn't working. A mack must not be in denial.

I recently got an e-mail from a guy that read:

Hey King Flex,
There is this girl that I have been trying to get with for the past three months. At first she seemed like she might be interested. But whenever we would try to set up a date or a hook-up, she would always flake out on me.

We used to talk on the phone a lot, but it seems like whenever I call her now, she is always in the middle of doing something else. Still, whenever I bring up the subject of hooking up, she always agrees that we should, but it never seems to materialize. How can I turn the tables on her, or at least get some

type of revenge on her for wasting my time by giving me the runaround for three months?
Signed,
"Fed Up"

And my response to him was:

Dear Fed Up,
Look, playa: The mackin' game isn't about revenge or vendettas. That's a waste of energy. Revenge is for super-heroes and Kung-Fu experts. The mackin' game is about tact and strategy. And if something isn't working for you, you have to take responsibility for it.

You have to accept the hand that you're dealt. If you and a particular female don't share the same vibe, don't waste three months of valuable mackin' time wondering why you and this female aren't working out or trying to fix it. Just charge that female to the game and keep it pimpin' else-where.

A lot of square guys are intrigued by the challenge of chasing a female and trying to wear her down until she gives in. But the mackin' game isn't about challenges, it's about cooperation.

I can understand a guy not wanting a serious relationship with a female who's too easy to get. Because if you got her too effortlessly, you think that other cats have gotten her just as ef-fortlessly. But a mack isn't going to break too much of a sweat trying to get with a female. And if something isn't working for you, switch up your techniques until you hit the jackpot.

If you're trying to move forward with your game, you can't keep bumping into a brick wall over and over, wishing that it wasn't there. You need to back up and take another route sometimes.

2) A mack must sometimes take his game on the road. A mack must not accept whatever is given to him.

I get an e-mail like this about once a month from different playas around the country:

Dear K-Flex,
It's very hard to find dimes or top-notch females in the city I live in. Most of the females here are hoodrats and chicken-heads.

Since there really isn't anything to do here in my city, all the females here seem to just get out of high school and have a gang of kids shortly thereafter. And the killing part is, all these hoodrats have stuck-up attitudes because all the guys are still trying to get at them.

Should I continue my seemingly endless journey to find top-notch females here, or should I just throw in the towel and settle for a chickenhead like all the other guys?
Signed,
"Small Town Player"

I tell guys like this that sometimes a mack has to pack it up and take the show on the road. As a mack, you should always have the drive, courage, and determination to set big goals, and make them happen. Even when it comes to getting dimes. There is nothing wrong with wanting to mack up on a top-notch female. Every man does. But because many guys have called it quits as far as upgrading their game in order to get a dime, they try to rationalize and justify being with lackluster females. ("She might be overweight, but at least she cooks good," or "She might be a chickenhead with four kids, but at least her Section 8 has put us in a nice crib," etc.)

The average man's basic goal in life is to try to stack as much paper as he can, and to get with a dime, or several. So if you are living in a city where your paper it isn't really growing and there are no tens, why stick around? Just move. Bounce. Raise up.

Some people might say, "Well, it costs money to relocate, and it's not easy to just up and leave." But there is a cost to be the boss. You can either settle for copper or upgrade to platinum.

When I was a kid, I moved from Detroit to Birmingham, Alabama. Birmingham is a great city now, and the people there are cool, but back in the eighties, it was hella slow. I mean real slow. Sometimes it even felt like time was going in reverse it was so slow. I remember feeling like I was in a mental prison when I lived there. I had already dated the few dimes that were down there at the time. There was no big money to be made. So at seventeen, I scraped up $125, purchased a one-way plane ticket to Los Angeles, and never looked back.

I didn't know anyone in Los Angeles and I didn't have a dime to my name, but I still pushed forward. Yes, I had to struggle for a while, but I felt that I had nothing to lose and everything to gain. To me, nothing could be worse than a life of mediocrity. I would rather struggle knowing I at least had the possibility of making a come-up (and I eventually did come up).

Now, there is nothing wrong with living the simple life if that's what you really want. But if you are unsatisfied with how you're living and where you're living, and you long to have better options when it comes to females, then you need to put on your thinking cap, lace up your pimp boots, and figure out a way to step to a better location. The same energy you use living in a small town and trying to make ends meet can be used in a better location to make millions. And the same energy you use to chase ducks you can use to get with dimes.

If your game isn't hitting in one city, I can almost guarantee that it will in the next. I'm not saying that you have to relocate to a major city to find females who are receptive to your game. I'm just saying you should try visiting different cities.

When you are on the campaign trail, you never know which city is going to have the most sympathetic "voters" who will feel your particular game. When I go on lecture tours, I sometimes take a few of the homies with me. We all have different personalities, and some guys get more play from the females in some cities than others. One of my partners, Frank, is a shirt-and-tie type of brother. In Dallas, it seemed like all the women there were giving him a lot of rhythm. I have another partner, Loc, who has that fresh-out-of-prison look, who is 100 percent gangsta. We went to Louisville, Kentucky, and the females went crazy over this cat. They were sweatin' Loc as if he were Usher or somebody, but many of them thought that Frank was too bougie.

I remember doing a lecture in Raleigh, North Carolina, and it seemed like every female I met there was a dime, and I've been to some cities where all the females look like stunt doubles for *Star Wars* movies. The point is, the mackin' game is sometimes regional and seasonal. You might be able to pull more women in Atlanta during the summertime than you would in New York during the winter.

If your game isn't working in one particular city, just remember that there are millions of females turning eighteen every day somewhere in this country. If you are in the right place at the right time, some of those females are going to choose you.

3) A mack must demand respect at all times. A mack must never let any form of disrespect go unchecked.

Even the most famous story in the Bible contains wisdom about mackin'. Adam was ordered by God not to eat fruit from a particular tree. Adam, who was supposed to be the leader of his relationship with Eve, instructed her that they were supposed to stay away, and not eat from the Tree of Knowledge. Not only did Eve, driven by her natural desire to rebel against male authority, eat from the tree anyway, but she convinced Adam to eat from it, as well. Instead of Adam checking Eve for disrespecting the game and going against his specific instructions, he let the situation go by unchecked, and ended up following his woman.

Even though it was Eve who influenced Adam to disobey God, Adam was specifically punished because it was his responsibility to be the leader in the relationship. Both Adam and Eve were punished by God for their disobedience.

This same dynamic is still going on to this day between men and women. Too many men are letting their women call the shots within the relationship. Too many men are following their women. Once a woman sees that she can boss you around, it's all downhill from there. No matter how docile, how submissive, how cool, or how sweet your female may be, sooner or later, she'll try to test you. All women want to push the boundaries with the men in their lives. And when women test you, you have to be mackish enough to stand up to the challenge.

Women have a natural tendency to rebel against male authority. It doesn't have to be for any particular reason. It's simply in their nature. This dynamic between men and women has existed since the beginning of time. Your woman might test you in a passive-aggressive way, or in a more blatant way. A woman might suddenly raise her voice to you in an inappropriate manner, and then monitor your reaction to it. She might tell you a blatant lie or purposely interact with an ex-boyfriend, and then sit back and study your response.

If a female sees that she can get away with a subtle form of disrespect, she will eventually try to get away with a more blatant form of disrespect. If you give her an inch, then next time she will take a mile. So as a mack, don't even give her a fraction of an inch. You have to check any form of disrespect at all times. When I say "check her," I don't mean beat her with clothes hanger. The best way to check a female is to let her know that you are a man with options, and that you don't have to accept any form of disrespect from her or any other woman.

The biggest trump card a mack can have is *options*. A mack must always be in a position (and make it clear to the females he is dealing with that he is in this position) to replace a female at any given moment. Like I said before, when some females see that they are a man's only dating option, they will have no reason to show a satisfactory level of respect. But when a female realizes that she can easily be replaced, she will mind her P's and Q's.

A lot of guys are afraid to check women who are disrespectful, because they don't want to jeopardize their poon-tang privileges. As a mack, you must never compromise your self-respect just for some coochie. Remember: Don't chase chicks, replace chicks.

4) A mack must look for, and train potential "stallions." A mack must not try to train "donkeys."

Here's another e-mail that I recently received, which represents a lot of other e-mails I've gotten from many brothers around the country;

Dear Tariq,

I'm a twenty-five-year-old mack-in-training, and I'm having problems with this older woman I'm dating. She is thirty-eight with three kids from previous relationships. As far as looks go, I would say she's about a six-and-a-half. She has a cute face, but she's a little chubby. The problem is, she's kind of bossy, and she insists on doing everything her way or no way. She's always bringing up problems she's had in past relationships, and we argue constantly. How do I turn the tables and become the shot-caller in the relationship? How do I get her in check and have her bow down to me instead of the other way around?

Signed,

"Frustrated Mack"

Dear Frustrated Mack (and all the other frustrated macks all over the world),

Let's take a close look at your situation: You are twenty-five years old. So your best mackin' years haven't even begun yet. And you are allowing yourself to be frustrated by a woman who is over ten years older than you, with three kids by different dudes, who talks to you crazy, and on top of all that, she's not even a dime (by your own admission)?

The real question is: Why even bother trying to get her mind right? What's the point? You need to charge her to the game and simply get with a female that's fresh off the lot, who's more qualified. It's like going out car shopping. Why waste time buying an old hooptie that you need to fix up, get smog-checked, put in a new engine, and worry about the mileage, when you can simply go out and spend the same amount of money getting a brand-new Lexus?

This is the difference between training a stallion and training a donkey. A young stallion is more valuable because it's strong, it's agile, it's in great physical shape, and it can be easily trained. After you train a young stallion, you can go out and win the Kentucky Derby or any other race with that stallion. And that stallion will remain loyal to you for a long time.

Now, a donkey is extremely stubborn. In order for you to get a donkey to do even minor tasks, you have to kick it, pull it, and beat it into submission. And even if you do finally break a donkey down and get it trained, what the hell are you going to do with a trained donkey, anyway? The whole frustrating process of training it is pointless.

This same analogy can be used when dealing with women. Why go through the headache of trying to get a female to be on the same wavelength as you, when she has a gang of psychological and emotional baggage, and she's not even a top-notch dime? Just go get a female who has yet to accumulate all that baggage.

Now I'm not trying to imply that all women over the age of thirty-five have a lot of baggage. Some women accumulate baggage at a very young age, as well. But on average, there are specific age groups of females who are less likely to have baggage than others.

From a general standpoint (and sure, there are exceptions) the best age group of females to get with are females between the ages of twenty-three and twenty-eight. During this period, women are getting out of the young hoochie stage, and they haven't quite reached the bitter, set-in-their-ways stage. During the twenty-three to twenty-eight period, women are very open-minded and receptive to the viewpoint of the men they date. So it is much easier to get one of these "stallions" to be on the same page you, as opposed to a bossy, bitter, "donkey" who has baggage left over from all of the other men she has dealt with in the past.

5) A mack must become fluent in nonverbal language. A mack must not accept everything at face value.

Like I mentioned before, over 90 percent of communication is nonverbal. So when you're mackin' on a female, the actual words she's saying to you are secondary. You should focus primarily on her body language and vocal inflections. And the best way to get a true assessment of a female is to see if her words match her body language. The problem with a lot of men is that they have been taught to trust everything a female tells them, and to take whatever a female tells them at face value. Society likes to perpetuate the myth that men are instinctive liars, and that women always tell the truth. But the reality is, many women are deceptive on an even deeper level than men are. When a man lies, he knows that he is full of it. But women's lies are more effective because women lie to *themselves.*

A lot of women are very convincing when they lie, because they believe their own BS. So as a mack, it's your job to decipher the nonverbal language. And once you get a true assessment of a female, you will be able to deal with her more effectively.

I've compiled a list of general terms, titles, and occupations that many women use to describe themselves. And I've also included the real meanings and translations of these titles. Here are a few:

Independent: . . . . .Woman who can't keep a man

Diva: . . . . .Woman over the age of thirty-five, woman over 150 lbs., or drag queen

Homemaker: . . . . .Baby mother who lives off a county check or a trick husband

Actress: . . . . .Waitress

Dancer: . . . . .Stripper

Masseuse: . . . . .Call girl

Makeup artist: . . . . .Girl who works in the cosmetic section at a department store

Real estate agent: . . . . .Female who is between jobs

Student (if under the . . .Female who is still living off her parents or age of twenty-three): student-loan money

Student (if over the . . . .Female who is still waiting on Captain Save-a-Ho age of twenty-three):

Stylist: . . . . .Hair dresser in the hood

Decorator: . . . . .Overweight girl or drag queen who is unemployed

Fashion designer: . . . . .Average-looking girl who is unemployed

Model: . . . . .Attractive female who is unemployed

6) A mack must use absence to increase desire. A mack must never allow himself to become too familiar or predictable.

A mack must always have an air of mystery. The less people—especially women—know about you, the better. When most guys meet women, they are too quick to divulge every bit of information about themselves. They think that by making a female aware of all of their credentials (real or made-up) they are impressing the female. This usually has the opposite effect. Once a female thinks you are trying to impress her, she will assume that she has something of value to you (usually it's her vagina). And a mack must always treat the vagina as if it has no value.

A mack must be as mysterious as possible. The less info you give about yourself, the more females will want to know about you. This is how you play to a woman's fantasies. The less you say about yourself and the more mysterious you are, the more women will project their fantasies and desires onto you. A mack should not be at a females beck and call at all times.

You have to initially let your presence (and good qualities) be known, and then you strategically make yourself scarce. You have to be purposely unpredictable. Always keep your female target enthralled with thoughts like, "I wonder where he is?", "I wonder what he's doing?", "I wonder what he's thinking about?", and "Is he thinking about me?" Your strategic absence, following a positive initial presence, will build up desire in a female.

When you're up in a female's face 24/7, and she pretty much

knows everything about you, she will look at you as being the average Joe Blow. But when you strategically remove yourself from a female's presence, and keep an air of mystery, you will come across as being larger than life. This is what's called the godlike effect. People are intrigued and obsessed by God because God is a total mystery to them. When Jesus walked the Earth like other men, he was crucified. But when he died leaving a promise of his return, people began to worship him.

There's an old saying: "Familiarity breeds contempt." People will easily project and attribute their failures, shortcomings, and frustrations onto the people who are around them on an everyday basis. In many cases, when you become a familiar fixture in a person's life, you will find yourself being a scapegoat for whatever goes wrong with that person. But when you strategically keep moving in and out of a female's presence, she will project only her positive desires and fantasies onto you. Once you've established this dominant yet mysterious, godlike presence, you will find that women will be willing to do anything for you.

The hit television show and movie *Charlie's Angels* utilized this concept. Charlie was a mysterious, unseen, godlike character whose "angels" (every God has his angels) were three female law-enforcement agents. Charlie would tell these women to do all types of dangerous tasks and missions all around the world, even though the angels had never even met Charlie in person.

You can have the same effect as long as you remain a puzzle to women. Once a female thinks she has an angle on you, switch your game up. Now don't confuse being mysterious with being deceitful. You don't have to lie about what you do or where you've been. I'm simply saying you should be vague about it and make yourself scarce sometimes. A mack has to be like a Picasso painting, vague and abstract. This way, women will try to interpret you in many different ways without getting a specific handle on you.

7) A mack must be bold in his decisions. A mack must never appear to be unsure or indecisive.

To be a mack, you must be a boss. As a matter of fact, if you look up the word *boss* in the dictionary, you will see many words that describe a true mack's personality (*Webster's Dictionary* defines the word *boss* as "a leader," and "a master," among other things). Like I said before, women instinctively look for leadership in men. To be a leader, you have to be extremely confident in your decision-making abilities. The reason why there aren't enough men who are leaders in their relationships today is because too many men are unsure of their agendas. A woman will not have confidence in a man's leadership if he isn't confident in his leadership ability first.

Bold decision-making is the easiest way to give off the appearance of confidence. Women don't respect indecisive men. Indecisiveness makes you look weak, and the essence of a mack is strength. Boldness will triumph over logic. All you have to do is appear as if you know what you're talking about. A bold, convincing execution will override any inconsistencies. If you can't win with wits, be bold with bullshit.

This is the philosophy that got president George W. Bush

reelected. There was a lot of evidence pointing out the Bush cabinet's inconsistencies and deceptive tactics in the war in Iraq. The hit movie *Fahrenheit 9/11* pointed this out and then some. Other presidential candidates who ran against Bush were more politically thorough and qualified for the position than he was. But Bush was so bold with his words and his decisions that it obscured all of his other inconsistencies. This is what helped him get so many votes.

When you establish a reputation for being bold and making definitive decisions, you won't have to check women as often. They will check themselves. Your boldness will make you seem unpredictable. People are always cautious about treading in unknown territory. Remember, you must be bold as well as tactful. Being bold isn't about being offensive. Running up to a female and saying, "Hey, you have nice titties," isn't being bold. That's being lame. You still must understand there is a time and place for everything. And your level of boldness should always be appropriate to the situation.

When you plan things with women, always take the initiative to be the captain of the team. You take her input into consideration, and then you make the final decision. If you are trying to plan a date with a female, and she asks, "What do you want to do?" don't reply with something indecisive like "I don't know. Whatever you want to do." You have to be a mack about it. Don't be afraid to call the shots. Tell her, "We are going to Roscoe's House of Chicken and Waffles, and then we will play it by ear," or something to that effect.

A major mistake that guys make when they first get with a female and don't quite have an angle on her yet is trying to brownnose their way into her good graces. This often backfires because it makes the guy come off as soft. The best way to get into the good graces of a female is to show her you have confidence. You do this with a bold, tactful presence. So when you deal with women, don't go out of your way to compromise.

Don't filibuster. Don't nitpick. And don't worry about being considered an asshole. It's better to be an asshole than an ass-kisser.

Top Five Accessories Macks Like to Sport

1. Pinky ring
2. Diamond-studded earrings
3. Rolex watch
4. Cuff links
5. Pimp cups

Top Five Accessories True Macks Do *Not* Sport

1. Anklet
2. Choker
3. Nipple ring
4. Tongue ring
5. Toe ring

8

ASS OR CASH?
GETTING WHAT YOU
REALLY WANT FROM FEMALES

Pop culture has always been secretly intrigued by the pimp game. And in recent years, this secret intrigue has become mainstream. This is due in part to the dominance of hip-hop culture. The pimp game was the precursor to hip-hop culture. If you read an Iceberg Slim book from the late 1960s (that talked about pimping in the 1920s and '30s) some of the exact slang terms from the book are used in hip-hop songs to this day. Back in the 1920s and '30s, pimps were into getting money, flashy cars, jewelry, and women. And almost every rap song and video out today is still about getting money, flashy cars, jewelry, and women.

Nowadays, many rappers are acknowledging the connection that hip-hop has to the pimp game. There are many rap songs about pimpin', and many songs that make references to pimpin'. And now many rappers are having actual pimps appear on their records and in their videos. Even though the flash and glitter of the pimp game has infiltrated the mainstream, the general public still has no idea about the true ins and outs of the game.

What's Your Real Agenda?

A lot of guys claim that they want to learn the pimp game because they want to have different females giving them gifts and money. But the reality is, many of these guys want to learn the pimp game because they figure this knowledge can help them have sex with a number of attractive females for free. Now if you are the kind of guy who is motivated by the prospect of having sex with a number of different women, there is nothing wrong with that. But you have to realize that this isn't pimping. In order to be in the pimp game, you must be sexually disciplined.

I would like to note that I'm not giving you this information so that you can go out and try to become an actual street pimp. Most guys who get into the game on a professional level were either born into the game or they got into the game out of necessity. If you have the option to choose another path in life, by all means do so. All the street players I know will be the first to tell you that the pimp game can be psychologically draining. In order for you to be successful in the game, you have to have the mental strength (and discipline) of ten men. But you should take heed to the basic principles of the pimpin' game. I feel there are lessons to be learned from the game that you can use in all walks of life.

Similarly, I wouldn't recommend that any person become a member of the Italian mafia. But I do admire some of the rules and codes mafia members observe. I believe that there are useful life lessons to be learned from every facet of society. What I'm trying to do in this section of the book is teach you some of the lessons from the pimp game that you can use in regular relationships with women. I want to do this without advocating pimpin' as a career or influencing anyone to totally embrace the whole pimp lifestyle.

Now if you're a cat who simply wants females to cater to him, bring him paper, and shower him with gifts, there is nothing wrong with that, either. You just have to be very honest with yourself and decide what's more important to you: ass or cash?

I know a lot of you guys are probably asking, "Well how come I can't have both?" "How come I can't have sex with different women all day, and get a lot of money from them in the process?" Because the game doesn't work that way. If you choose one, you sacrifice the other to a small degree.

Many guys want to get into the pimpin' game because they are sex freaks who are addicted to poon-tang, but you cannot be a freak *and* a pimp. That's like a drug dealer who smokes crack. And you can't sex your way up on some big money from females. Sexing females for money makes you a gigolo. And gigolo money isn't the same as pimp money.

The Difference Between a Pimp and a Gigolo

Guys who get money and gifts from females generally get labeled as pimps. There are guys who have the ability to get a couple of bucks out of a few females, who think they are pimpin'. But in reality, most of these guys are just gigolos.

The gigolo game and the pimp game are totally different. In the gigolo game, the man is exchanging sexual favors for gifts and money from females. In the pimp game, the man is exchanging game for money. There is basically one way that a man can be considered a pimp. The only way to be a pimp is if you have a prostitute, call girl, escort, or stripper who gets money from tricks, on a nightly basis, and then brings the money to you. If you are not doing this, then you are not a pimp. Everything else, as far as getting money and gifts from females, falls under the gigolo category instead.

Pimps get money from hos. Gigolos get money from square females. In the pimp game, the man is in total control of the women. This is because he depends on his game and not his women. And his game will help him recruit a number of different females in case one of his women decides to dip. But in the gigolo game, the female is in control. This is because the gigolo depends on the female. And if a female decides to cut him loose, he is assed-out. There are three main types of gigolo. They are:

1. The High-Stakes Gigolo
2. The Down-on-His-Luck Gigolo
3. The Low-Budget Gigolo

Here is an assessment of all of the three types:

The High-Stakes Gigolo

These are the professional gigolos who know how to go after the big fish. Many High-Stakes Gigolos work with professional escort agencies that hire them out as companions to women. Many of these guys attend upper-class events in order to scout for their targets.

Many High-Stakes Gigolos also work as male exotic dancers in order to supplement their income, as well as to recruit sugar mamas. These types of gigolos are usually well groomed and they tend to be very physically fit. They place a lot of emphasis on their bodies, because they are essentially selling sex to women. The main demographic of women who need to pay a man for sex and companionship on a regular basis are older women and overweight women. These are the High-Stakes Gigolo's primary targets.

These guys primarily target older women (especially widows) because, for the most part, many older women are the only women with disposable income that they can trick off. Many High-Stakes Gigolos are bisexual. Unlike most heterosexual men, many High-Stakes Gigolos have no problem with sexing up an elderly female. If a guy like this can have sex with another man, he really wouldn't have too much of a problem with having sexual intercourse with an elderly or morbidly overweight female. If you need more proof of this, just look at all of the older female celebrities who have gotten married to younger men. If you take a close look at these husbands, they all seem a little "suspect."

Most young heterosexual men couldn't be High-Stakes Gigolos. Unlike young women who manage to have sex with elderly men for money, straight men find it extremely difficult to have sex with elderly women, no matter how much money they have. *You can't bribe your dick*. Either a man is sexually turned-on by a female or he's not. But the High-Stakes Gigolo can hang out with a physically unattractive female with no problem. This type of guy likes to hang out with older women and do "girlie" things with them. They go shopping together. They go to the ballet together. They go to shoe stores together. The High-Stakes Gigolo is willing to do all the things that the average straight guy wouldn't be caught dead doing.

The Down-on-His-Luck Gigolo

This type of gigolo likes to use the sympathy approach on his female targets. He likes to seem like the good guy who is just trying to get back on his feet. The Down-on-his-Luck Gigolo usually targets square females within his own age group.

He will come into a woman's life with a gentlemanly approach, appearing as if he's got himself together. But once he gets his foot in the door with a female, he will conveniently "lose his job," "get evicted," "have his car put in the shop," etc. When the woman he is dealing with sees this, her maternal instincts kick in and she helps him out. The Down-on-his-Luck Gigolo is a master of getting females to invest in one of his "dreams," which he knows will never pay off.

The Down-on-his-Luck Gigolo doesn't bring in the type of money that the High-Stakes Gigolo brings in. This is because the Down-on-his-Luck Gigolo focuses on younger women with square jobs. These females don't usually have the disposable income that can mean big money.

The Low-Budget Gigolo

This is the type of gigolo who specializes in targeting welfare queens and hoodrats. The Low-Budget Gigolo has very low expectations, and he looks for women who can provide him with basic living necessities.

Many of these types of gigolos become professional baby-daddies. These guys will go out and find a number of hoodrats who are willing to have babies with them. Then they live off these women.

Low-Budget Gigolos grew up in inner-city, single-mother homes. They are used to having dominating women in their lives, so they seek out these mother/child relationships with other women when they become adults.

Since these guys really have no tight game (if they did, would they be shacking up with females in the projects?) they have to use sex as their only bargaining chip. These guys are totally dependent on the females they deal with. They depend on the female to buy them clothes, let them borrow her car, and even buy them the discs for their Xboxes (many Low-Budget Gigolos love sitting up in women's homes all day playing Xbox). The ironic thing about Low-Budget Gigolos is that these are the main cats who like to go around bragging about how much they are big-pimpin'.

If It's Ass that You Desire . . .

Now, if your primary goal when you meet women is to get some quick and easy ass, there are techniques to help you accomplish this. First you have to at least be honest with yourself and acknowledge that this is your primary goal. And you must understand that you don't have to exert an unnecessary amount of energy and time just to get some ass from a female.

A lot of men will exert an unnecessary amount of energy on a female they really aren't into in order to compensate for the guilt felt over just wanting sex. If all you want to do is get sex from a female, there are three simple techniques you can use. They are:

1. The Earn/Reward Method
2. The Mysterious Mack Method
3. The Bold-Faced Lie Method

The Earn/Reward Method

The Earn/Reward Method is when you meet a female and you get her to invest something in you. When a man goes on a date with a female and invests in drinks, dinner, movies, etc., at the end of the date, he wants a payoff, usually sex.

Women are the same way. When a female is required to invest in a man, she wants a payoff, as well. But usually the payoff she wants is a commitment of some sort. But most men don't require a female to invest anything. So they can't fathom the idea of a female willingly bringing something to the table.

A professional pimp understands this dynamic. This is how a lot of pimps hook their females. You have to establish early on with a female that she has to bring something else to the table besides sex. You have to give a female chores. You have to make her cook for you. You have to require her to come over and clean your crib. You have to require her to take you out. You have to require her to run errands for you.

You have to make her earn your affection. What you will see happen is that she will start trying to give you sex just to get out of doing so many chores. As a mack, you use sex as a reward to her. In order to use this technique, you have to be very disciplined. If you do it correctly, this technique can be used over an extended period of time with a female.

The Mysterious Mack Method

The Mysterious Mack Method is when you become a secretive, ambiguous figure in the eyes of a female. This way, you will tap into the woman's fantasies and allow her to project her desires onto you.

This technique works best when you step to females from areas other than where you live. It won't work if the female is familiar with where you are from and the people you hang out with. Contrary to popular belief, most women have had one-night stands. But they will never admit to this, because they don't want to be perceived as stanks.

Many adult females have had a secret sexual encounter at least once with a mysterious guy that they knew little about. The fact that the man was so mysterious is the reason the woman can keep the encounter a secret. Some women might even block the encounter out of their minds. Some females fantasize about the encounter all the time. Nonetheless, you need to become one of these mysterious macks.

This is by far the easiest way of getting quick, easy, commitment-free sex from females. All you have to do is pop up in a club or social spot where people don't know your face, and then start stepping to females on a courtesy level without revealing too much about yourself. You have to reveal all your best personal qualities (such as being well groomed, nicely dressed, extremely confident) without coming across like you're flossing. All you have to do is keep your mouth shut, stay cool, be very vague about yourself, don't reveal too much, and allow yourself to become a blank canvas.

This way, you can allow a female to paint whatever picture she wants about you. When women first meet a man who they can project their fantasies onto, they get into a somewhat euphoric, hypnotic state. So it's very important to position yourself to get the ass within four days of meeting a female when using the Mysterious Mack Method. If you wait too long, the hypnotic spell will wear off. And the longer you wait to get the ass, the more difficult it will become.

The Bold-Faced Lie Method

Now the Bold-Faced Lie Method for getting sex is the only circumstance in the mackin' game in which I condone lying. Contrary to popular belief, the mackin' game is really about honesty and fairness. As you may have noticed, no other part of this book has suggested using deception toward women. But I do condone lying when it comes to getting superficial, one-night-stand sex. I do not condone the Bold-Faced Lie Method if you are trying to establish an ongoing relationship with a female. Again, out of respect for the game, you should only use this technique if you are trying to get some quick, one-night-stand sex.

You go to a club or a social event in a city or location where no one knows you. And when you meet females there, simply lie about your occupation. When you lie, don't tell a half-assed lie. If you are going to lie, you might as well go all-out with it. As a matter of fact, the bigger the lie, the more believable it will seem.

If the female asks what you do for a living, tell her that you are a professional athlete. Tell her that you are a prince from an African country. Tell her you're an architect. Tell her you just bought the BET Network. Tell her you are the new road manager for G-Unit. Tell her that you just purchased two Popeye's Chicken franchises in the area. Tell her that you are a video director.

Remember, the bigger and bolder the lie, the better. I can almost guarantee you if you go to a club where no one knows who you are, and you tell enough bold lies (like the ones I mentioned) to a number of females, one of them will be down to sex you up that night. And if a female is superficial enough to have sex with you because she thinks that you are a professional athlete, or that you own a Popeye's Chicken franchise, then you should be superficial enough to tell bold-faced lies about what you do. This is why I only condone lying under these circumstances.

Twelve Things a Mack Would Never Say to Get Sex

1. "I love you." (The *extreme* bold-faced lie approach)
2. "If you really cared about me, you would do it." (The guilt-trip approach)
3. "Take off your clothes so I can give you a massage." (The "I'm hooking *you* up" approach)
4. "Let me just put the *head* in." (The bargaining approach)

5. "I normally don't have sex on the first date either, but you're special." (The brownnosing approach)
6. "I'll buy you anything you want." (The trick's approach)
7. "I just *got* to have you." (The sympathy approach)
8. "There are a bunch of other girls who would love to do it with me." (The egotistical approach)
9. "Okay, then just go down on me." (The Bill Clinton approach)
10. "I just want to put it in and take it right back out." (The "let me sample it" approach)
11. "Let's just take off our clothes. We don't have to do nothing." (The "take my word for it" approach)
12. "You want a ride home, don't you?" (The hostage approach)

If It's Cash You Desire . . .

As I explained before, there are only two mentalities that a man can have: a pimp mentality, or a trick mentality. Some of the most successful people in the world with leadership positions (from hustlers to executives to CEOs, etc.), were born with a pimp mentality. If you were not born with a pimp mentality, you can acquire this mentality through strong discipline. When it comes to recruiting females who can bring something to the table besides sex, it is imperative that you have a pimp mentality.

The first step in recruiting females who can bring things to the table is learning how to trump the pussy card. This is extremely hard for the average man to do. In order to be a thorough mack, you must have a "purse first, ass last" mentality.

Here is a test you can take that will determine what type of mentality you have. Just imagine this: If someone were to offer you $10,000 (not a whole hell of a lot of money, but a fairly nice amount of paper) to sleep in the same bed with Halle Berry every night for one month, but not have sex with her, no matter how much she comes on to you, could you do it?

Now be honest with yourself. Ten Gs, or a piece of Halle Berry? Think about that, fellas. Halle is fine as hell. And ten Gs. You can do a lot with ten Gs. Master P started No Limit Records, which is now worth hundreds of millions of dollars, with a $10,000 investment. So there *are* ways you can move and shake with ten Gs.

I think given a choice between ten grand and sex with Halle Berry, the average man would start tearin' that pussy up within two days. Any cat who is sexually disciplined enough to trump the pussy card and hold out for the $10,000 definitely has a pimp mentality. This is the dilemma that professional pimps go through every single day. They have to constantly trump pussy cards all the time, if they want to get any kind of money.

As I mentioned before, when you require females to bring something to the table, they will try to use sex as a bargaining chip to wiggle their way out of doing their chores for you. If your main objective is to get money, you must never allow your woman to use sex as a bargaining chip. Once you do that, she will view you as just a trick.

Finding Females with the Means to Break Bread

The first step to recruiting females who will break bread is finding a female who has disposable paper. I know we often hear females saying things like, "I will never give a man money, blah, blah, blah." But in most cases, females who say this have no money to give, anyway.

The reality is that women who have a significant amount of paper are glad to give it to men they are into. The majority of young, attractive women (especially women in their late teens to mid-twenties) who have this type of disposable income are women who are in the game.

Let's face it, if you meet a twenty-one-year-old female who is living in a tight crib on her own, driving a fly whip, and sporting high-end gear, either she's living off of a trust fund, or she has some hoin' under her belt. There aren't too many females living off trust funds in this country. But there *is* a whole lot of hoin' going on. The only way to step to a female who is living a professional-ho lifestyle is to have a pimp mentality.

Know Your Ho

A very important rule of the game is knowing what type of ho you are dealing with. People in the game put women into two general categories: squares and hos.

Now, the majority of what you have read in this book so far has been about how to deal with what we call "square" females. You have to deal with hos a little differently. First you have to know the basic definition of what a ho is. Often, people equate a ho with a prostitute. But there is a difference. A *ho* is a female who has sex with two or more people within a one-month time span. A *prostitute* is a female who has sex with two or more people within a one-month time span and gets paid for it.

A lot of people think the label of *ho* comes into play because of the exchange of money. But the *ho* tag is based on having multiple sex partners. Now I'm sure there are people out there who will start whining about the so-called double standard, and say things like, "What about a man who has multiple sex partners? Aren't these men considered hos, too?"

My answer to them is yes, some men are hos, too. But the difference between a male ho and a female ho is that a male ho has no problem admitting to his hoishness. A man can sleep with five females in one week, then wake up the next day, look in the mirror, and pop his collars to himself. But if the average female sleeps with five guys in a week, she will most likely try to block it out of her mind, be in denial about it, or come up with excuses about it: "I was drunk," "I was vulnerable," "I think I was drugged," etc.

The point is, most female hos (professional or non-pro) will not admit to being hos. So you first have to determine whether or not the female you are dealing with is a ho, and then you have to figure out what type of ho she is.

There are a few different categories of hos. A female who dresses very skimpily and provocatively to get attention is called a *hoochie*. A female who has sex with a number of men (and women) just because she enjoys a lot of sexual contact with different people, is called a *slut*. A female who has sex with a number of men in exchange for menial items (such as food, weed, drinks, clothes, trips to the nail shop, etc.) is called a *stank*. A female who has sex in exchange for a set price is called a *hooker*.

A female who has limited sexual contact with different tricks, whose price range varies and who sells her companionship, is called a *call girl*. A female who gets money by spitting game at different guys without actually having sex with them is called a *hustler*. A female who has sex for money and still gets paid years after she stops having sex, is called a *wife*.

Pro-Hos

If you are trying to step to females using a pimp mentality, you need to step to pro-hos. Pro-hos fall into the category of hookers, strippers, and call girls. The problem is trying to differentiate between real hos and females who are just hoish. Many females who act hoish just for the attention will display over-the-top behavior when they go out. These attention freaks usually hang out with other attention freaks. Their main goal when they go out is to be seen.

Most pro-hos are very low-key when they are outside of their work environment. They almost go out of their way to appear conservative. But there are a few clues to look for in a female to help you tell if she is in the game. The four signs to look for to tell if a female might be a ho:

1. If she wears a tongue ring or any other type of facial piercing.
2. If she wears a lot of blue eye shadow.

3. If she is hanging out in the club by herself. (Most women in the game are hated on by square females, and pro-hos know how scandalous other pro-hos can be, so they just tend to go out by themselves.)
4. If she has three or more visible tattoos.

Now of course there are exceptions to the rule, but generally when you find a female with one or more of these four characteristics, she just might have a foot in the game and some ho stripes on her sleeve.

When you are dealing with a female who is in the game, you have to establish very quickly that you are not a man who can be manipulated sexually. Because a woman who is in the game will quickly test any man she comes into contact with.

These women are used to dominating and manipulating men every day. So you have to have a boss mentality and stand up to any test these women might spring up on you. The hardest part of getting females to break bread is screening through all the broke females and the decoy hos, in order to get to the qualified females. And once you finally get with a female in the game who is qualified to break bread, all you have to do is sit back and be mackish.

All women have an insatiable need for companionship. And this is especially true for women in the game. It's so difficult for women in the game to sustain meaningful, significant relationships—when most guys step to women in the game, they are either trying to pay for sex, or they're trying to hustle up some free sex—that these women have a stronger need for real companionship. That's what a pimp, boss player, or true mack provides: companionship for women in the game.

There is one basic, simple rule that you must understand when you are dealing with women in the game, or females who have paper. If she likes you, she will pay you.

Top Five Greatest Gigolos of All Time

1. Stedman Graham
2. Kevin Federline
3. Chris Judd
4. Al Reynolds
5. Bobby Brown

9

UPGRADING YOUR GAME

After my first book, *The Art of Mackin'*, came out, I got lots of e-mails from readers, and most of them were asking the same questions. But there was one e-mail that really, really moved me. This one guy wrote me and said that he once had such a lack of confidence when it came to getting with women that he would use heavy drugs and alcohol in order to get a false sense of confidence. As a result, he eventually became a serious drug addict. He told me that reading *The Art of Mackin'* had taught him how to have real self-confidence. And he said that the book motivated him to check into a drug rehab facility and turn his life around.

I was particularly moved by this letter because I appreciated seeing that this guy fully understood what the mackin' game is truly about. The mackin' game isn't just limited to getting females. Once you fully understand the rules and the nature of the mackin' game, you can upgrade your game and apply it to everything in your life.

Mackin' in the Business World

One of the biggest macks in the business world is Donald Trump. Whenever you see Donald Trump, he is always chillin' with a supermodel. He has put himself into a position to get the best women on the market. And he uses the same mack mentality when he conducts his business deals.

Trump knows how to promote his name. He knows how to schmooze his targets. He knows how to use charisma and charm to close deals. And he knows how to quickly dismiss anyone who doesn't approach him with respect. This is what has made him one of the most successful businessmen in the country.

You have to treat every life endeavor, whether it's a business endeavor, academic endeavor, social endeavor, etc., as if it were a female you are trying to recruit. When you're dealing with a female, you have to let her know that you are in demand. This makes you appear to be more valuable to her. And when you are trying to close a business deal, you have to let your business associates know that you are in demand.

When you deal with females, you can't seem too eager to get with them. You have to play it cool. In the same way, when you are trying to close a business deal, you also can't seem overly eager. Appearing overly eager makes you seem suspicious, whether you are dealing with females or business associates.

The point is, you've got to learn how to parlay the game you use to spit at females into other aspects of your life. The way you mack is a reflection of your overall character. The way a man handles his females should reflect the way he handles all of his other life and business endeavors.

Your Game Reflects Your Character

If you have a reputation for lying, cheating, and deceiving females you date, people will assume that you will lie, cheat, and deceive in general. They will be reluctant to do business with you. If you are true to the game and straight-up (no matter how big a player you are) in the way you deal with women, people are more likely to respect your character.

This doesn't mean you can't get any. Again, look at Donald Trump. Trump changes women like he changes draws, and makes no secret of it. And this hasn't affected the level of respect he gets as a businessman. Hugh Hefner admits to having seven girlfriends in his stable, and Hef is highly respected in this country. When Bill Clinton admitted to having sexual relations with Monica Lewinsky, his approval rating with the American public was unaffected. Now *that's* a mack.

In contrast, let's look at someone like Scott Peterson. Scott Peterson was accused of killing his pregnant wife, Laci Peterson. The physical evidence linking him to the murder was minimal. But when the prosecution revealed that he cheated on his wife and was deceptive in the way he dealt with his mistress, people automatically assumed that he was deceptive about everything else, including the murder—and he was convicted.

Remember to have integrity with your game, because this will enhance your overall reputation and character. Always leave a positive impression with the people you deal with on an intimate, social, or business level.

Other Mack Upgrades

The majority of this book has dealt primarily with the overall mentality a man must have to be a true mack. But a mack must also look the part, so now I would like to point out a few accessories a mack can use to upgrade his status. Let's start with:

Jewelry

When it comes to jewelry, we are in an age where it's best to be subtle. Back in the seventies and eighties, it was fly to walk around sporting huge gold chains and four finger rings. But now, less is more.

When you get suited and booted, it is always good to finish off the ensemble with something that sparkles. A pinky ring. A nice watch. Nice cuff links or a nice necklace. Women have a natural attraction to things that glitter, and jewelry helps you send a message that you have something of a flair to your personality.

Hair

This should go without saying, but a mack's hair should be on-deck at all times. I have to mention this because I have seen guys going out to clubs with "unestablished" hairlines and fuzzy braids.

When you're trying to put your mack down, you have to give females the impression that you take pride in your looks. This is not possible if your hair looks like you've been wearing a football helmet. Spend the money to get your hair lined up, player. Take time out to get your braids redone. When your dome is looking right, you will have a better self-image.

Remember to keep your hairstyles current. Don't walk off in the club sporting a Bobby Brown "My Prerogative" gumby from 1988. And this goes for all of my white macks out there, as well. I've seen a few of you white cats out there in the clubs with your hair feathered. Unless you are part of a Bee Gees cover band, switch your 'do up. And chill out with the mullets. Mullets and mackin' *cannot* coexist. A true mack should keep his hair in an up-to-date, well-groomed style. And remember, the only time you should rock a perm is if you are doing some full-fledged pimpin'.

Shoes

Shoes are crucial for completing the look of a top-notch mack. Many guys are unaware of this, but the first thing a woman notices on a man is his shoes. Women understand how shoes say a lot about someone's personality, because they are shoe experts. This is why they approach shoe-shopping like an art form. Women take pride in the shoes they buy for themselves, because they understand how shoes send out a nonverbal message about the person wearing them. So when women first meet a man, they look at his shoes to see what nonverbal message he is sending about himself.

You always want to have shoes that send the message that you are a mack. To a mack, the shoes are the most important part of his clothing ensemble. The wrong shoes can totally ruin a good outfit. So always take pride in your footwear and the message it sends. Here are a few examples of the different types of shoes men wear, and the nonverbal message they send to women:

SHOES	NONVERBAL MESSAGE
Sneakers	"I have a little youth in me."
Timberland boots	"I've got a little thug in me."
Alligator shoes	"I have a little player in me."
Hush Puppies	"I have a little geek in me."
Flip-flops	"I have a little hippie in me."
Sandals	"I'm married."
Cowboy boots	"I have a little hillbilly in me."
Mules	"I have a little queen in me."

Keeping Your Game on a Certain Level After You Upgrade

When you reach third-degree mack status, you must always maintain a level of integrity that will keep you at the top of your game. This is because mackin' is also about maintenance. Making a million dollars is a task. But maintaining that million dollars after you make it is another task within itself. And in the mackin' game, upgrading your convo, grooming habits, clothing, and shoes is one major task. Maintaining this level of game is something you have to constantly work at, as well.

There are two general areas of game maintenance that a true mack must uphold when dealing with women. They are:

1. Booty-Call Etiquette
2. Pussy-Whipping Immunity

Booty-Call Etiquette

When it comes to booty calls, many men tend to let their standards drop. Men usually start off the evening with hopes of a high-level booty call, but since most booty calls are spontaneous, most guys will settle for whatever booty is available to them when they want it. The general rule for the average man, as far as booty calls go, is that the later it gets, the lower the standards go.

When it's early in the evening, the average guy gets out his cell phone and starts off trying to contact the top-grade females. When it gets a little later in the evening, he starts breaking out with the little black book of females he keeps in touch with from time to time. And when those females aren't available, he starts dusting off that old, little black book that's buried in the back of the closet. (All guys have been reduced to digging in that old phone book at one point or another. Guys, you know what I'm talking about: the little black book you've had since the "Please Hammer Don't Hurt 'Em" tour of '91.)

At around seven or eight p.m., you start calling up the Halle

Berry- and Tyra Banks-looking females. At around nine or ten p.m., guys start downgrading and calling up the Naomi Campbell and the Alicia Keys females. At around eleven or midnight, the females start looking like Pamela Anderson. After midnight, the females start looking like Louie Anderson.

When you reach true mack status, you never let it get to that point. Always limit how low you will let your standards drop when campaigning for a booty call. A booty call female should be no lower than a six (by your own standards of what a six is). When you get desperate, and start calling fives and twos, you send a negative message about yourself to your subconscious mind. It's like telling yourself that you don't deserve better. So always maintain proper Booty-Call Etiquette and keep your mack standards intact.

Pussy-Whipping Immunity

In order for a true mack to maintain his third-degree status, he must become immune to being pussy-whipped. As I stated before, the average man's weakness is in being sexually manipulated by women. Once you have elevated and upgraded your game to the point where you are immune to a woman's pussy-whipping tactics, you will feel the full power of total mackdom.

The worst type of pussy-whipped man is a guy who doesn't realize he's whipped. As I mentioned in the beginning of this book, there are a few ways to determine whether or not you are whipped. So I'm going to give you a test that will help you determine if you are pussy-whipped. If two or more of the ten items on the test applies to you, then you are a certified pussy-whipped brother. If you fail this test, I suggest that you put this book down, go rent *The Di-*

vine Secrets of the Ya-Ya Sisterhood, and go chill with the female that whipped you.

Top Ten Ways to Know If You're Whipped

1. If your lady gives you a curfew, and you abide by it
2. If you baby-sit a female's kids (who aren't yours) while she goes out to the club
3. If you get a female's name tattooed on your arm
4. If you go out in public wearing matching outfits with your female
5. If you carry your lady's purse at the mall
6. If you call up radio stations to dedicate songs to your lady
7. If your lady makes you sit through chick flicks on a regular basis
8. If you have ever uttered the words, "I don't want to lose you" to a female
9. If you have ever dropped out of school or quit a job over a female
10. If you have ever found yourself standing in the grocery store checkout line with a bottle of Summers Eve or a box of Tampax

If you are a pussy-whipped brother, the best thing for you to do is shake that pussy vice cold turkey. Refuse to let the coochie control your life. Start recruiting other females so you won't feel forced to focus on that one coochie that has your mind.

You should also become hip to some of the tactics women use to test you. One of the most common ways women test men is by trying to send them on errands. The errand might start off small, at first. It might seem innocent and minute, initially. But if she can get away with having you run a small errand, the next time it will be a bigger one. If you are always willing to run every errand that a woman requests, she will know that she has you whipped.

Every man out there has experienced this scenario before: You are on your way over to a female's crib to kick it with her when she calls you up and says something like, "Hey, can you stop by Baskin-Robbins and pick up some ice cream for me before you come by?" This might seem like an innocent request, but in reality it is a test.

If you haven't had sex with a female yet and she asks you to run an errand like this, she either A) wants to test you to see how badly you want to hit it, or B) is already planning on getting busy with you, and wants to give her conscience the impression that she made you earn the privilege of having sex with her.

If you *have* already had sex with a female and she is trying to get you to run errands for her, she is definitely trying to see if she has you pussy-whipped. As far as the rules of the mackin' game, you are allowed to run only one mirror errand for a female you just hooked up with, or better yet, none at all.

If a female is clearly testing you by trying to make you stop and pick up some items for her on your way over to her crib, you need to mack up and say *hell no*. Tell her if she wants somebody to bring food to her crib she needs to call Meals-on-Wheels. Don't ever let a female think she has you pussy-whipped by running errands and picking up food for her.

Now if the female is down to do the same for you, then it's cool to reciprocate. If you are doing all the running and she is doing all the chillin', then she's going to feel like she has you whipped. That's when you need to shake that pussy vice off you and give her the number to Domino's for when she gets hungry.

After that, start building up your pussy immune system, so the only time you will go to the grocery store for a female is when you are picking up some Lawry's Season Salt so she can spice up the meal *she* is cooking for *you*.

Tips on Setting the Right Tone

Another very important mack upgrade is learning how to set the right tone when a female comes over to your crib. When you invite a female over to your spot for the first time, your general goal is to hit it. In order to increase the possibility of this, you need to make females comfortable when they're in your home. One way to do this is to put on the right music.

Obviously, you shouldn't have a female over when your crib is filthy. No matter how good the music is, a female isn't going to be comfortable with roaches crawling on her. You should also have the right lighting (the good ol' red lightbulb is a player's classic) and the right scent. Don't invite a woman over to your place with your crib smelling like chicken grease and ass. Light a scented candle and spray some Febreze on your bedsheets, homie. With the basics covered, nice music and, in some cases, nice drinks, are the best icebreakers when you have a female over.

Types of Music to Play

Music brings out all types of passions and emotions in people. Some songs bring out anger or aggressiveness. There are some songs that come on in the club and make people want to fight. Some songs bring out sadness. Some songs bring out joy. So it's understandable that some music will bring out other human emotions, such as sexual desire and comfort.

A mack's music has to be appropriate for the female he is with. If you are with a younger female, say between eighteen and twenty-one, you might want to start off with some hip-hop, and then after she gets in her comfort zone, slow it down with some Alicia Keys, or something similar.

If it's an herbal-tea type of female (you know, the bohemian type) you definitely need to break out with the Jill Scott and the Erika Badu. If you have a more sophisticated female, you can't go wrong with a little jazz music. Whatever music you need to get your females in their comfort zones, you need to hook it up. Just remember, don't play the wrong type of music for the wrong type of female. You can't invite a female from the 'hood over to your crib and try getting her in the mood by playing Kenny G. And you can't woo a top-notch, sophisticated female by playing the remix to "Move Bitch, Get Out the Way."

One minor slip-up can potentially get a woman out of her comfort zone with you and salt your whole game up. If you are unsure what type of music to play around your female, you can't go wrong with the Isley Brothers. Any slow cut from the Isley Brothers will set the mood.

I have one CD that is one of my personal favorites to get females in a mellow mood when they come over to the crib. It's the first CD from the R&B group 112, self-titled *112*. Almost every one of the nineteen songs on the CD are slow cuts. Every time I put that CD on when a female comes by my crib, her panties start dropping like stock prices. You can just put that 112 CD on, and let it ride all night.

If you have a CD burner, you should compile a number of songs with suggestive lyrics that will send subtle messages and innuendo to the female who is coming to see you. The songs should be in a certain sequence depending on what message you want to send to the female at any particular time. Here are a few examples of five songs you should burn onto your booty-call CD:

1. "Do Me Baby" by Prince
2. "There's a Meeting in My Bedroom" by Silk
3. "Turn Off the Lights" by Teddy Pendergrass
4. "Bump and Grind" by R. Kelly

And after you finish getting your freak on:

5. "Hit the Road, Jack" by Ray Charles

How to Avoid Spending Money on Dates

Fellas, are you tired of going out on dates you really don't want to go on, and spending money you really don't want to spend when dealing with females? Well here is a game-spitting technique I like to call the King Flex Method that you can use to help get you out of an unwanted date situation. In order to master this technique, you have to prepare yourself for a mental chess game. Most square guys have a checkers-game mentality. In checkers, your job is to jump on whatever opportunity is available. Most square guys will accept anything a female throws their way. This is why their females usually end up with the upper hand. But a true mack must think like a chess player. You have to be two steps ahead of the opposing player at all times.

When you use the King Flex Method on females, you will be able to get females to say what you want them to say by thinking ahead. If you use the King Flex Method correctly, not only will you avoid money coming out of your pockets, you will also have females taking *you* out on dates. The only time you will have to go into your pockets is to get a condom.

It works like this: When you first meet a female and you have your initial phone conversation, you start mentioning how you would like to meet a female who is really independent. Talk about how so many women claim to be independent but they really aren't. This will make your female target start bragging about how independent she is. We have all heard the "I'm independent" speech from women before, so you should already be familiar with this.

You want to prompt her to continue bragging about how independent she is by saying things like, "Sure, you say you're independent, but you might be just like all the other females out there who say they're independent. When it comes time to bring something to the table, they fall short." This will make her determined to separate herself from all the other females who say they are independent. She is really going to want you to buy her "independent woman" claims. So you say something like, "Let me throw a hypothetical situation at you. Let's say you and I were dating. Or let's just say you were dating any guy, for that matter. What can you bring to the table? What is the incentive for a guy to be in a relationship with you?"

Notice how I threw in that "any guy, for that matter." If you just ask her, "If I were dating you, what could you bring to the table?" all she would do is avoid the question with another question: "Well, what can *you* bring to the table?" But when you mention the scenario of her dating guys in general, she is forced to answer the question. She'll run down a list of what she can do and what she can bring to the table in a relationship, and when she's done, that's when you go in for the kill. You say to her (in a very smooth, mellow, and non-condescending way) "Ok, well you definitely are independent. And since you are so independent, why don't you take me out to dinner tomorrow night?" Now, 98 percent of all women have never had a guy ask them that before, so this will throw her off-balance, which is what you want. And in any game, when your opponent is off-balance, you have the upper hand.

When you ask a woman to take you out on a date, I can all but guarantee that she will come back with one of these three replies:

1. "Why don't you take *me* out on a date?"
2. "I don't take guys out on dates first."
3. "I'm old-fashioned, and I believe that men should take women out."

Now if she says, "Why don't you take *me* out on a date?" or "I don't take guys out first," she knows she is contradicting all that stuff she just said about being independent. So most females will agree to take you out on a date just to save face. When the female says that she is still old-fashioned when it comes to dating, you say to her, "Cool, I like old-fashioned women. So since you are so old-fashioned, why don't you come over to my crib and cook for me? That's what women did in the old days."

If you break it down like that, the female will most likely agree to cook dinner for you or take you out on a date. I have been using this method for years, and it always works like a charm. Remember, when you use this technique, you have to back it up with confidence. Don't worry about jeopardizing your chances of having sex with a female. Trust me, she will respect your confidence if she's real about hers.

Top Five Most Famous Pussy-Whipped Men of All Time

1. Will Smith: Being henpecked isn't too bad if you are pecked by the right hen. Will's current wife, Jada Pinkett-Smith, is the right hen. So you still get player points, Will. But you still need some points deducted because you put yourself in a position to let your first wife take you to the cleaners.
2. Doug Christie: NBA player whose wife follows the team bus in her own car in order to keep an eye on him.
3. Mike Tyson: During his Robin Givens period.
4. John Wayne Bobbitt: His wife cut his jimmy off, and he still wanted to work things out.
5. J. Howard Marshall: This was the old Texas billionaire who had one foot in the grave and another foot in the strip club when he met Anna Nicole Smith.

CONCLUSION

The main thing I hope you have learned from this book is how to have respect. When I say "have respect," I mean have respect for yourself first. If you don't respect yourself, and you feel that you are inferior to the females you are trying to get with, there it is no way you can truly respect others.

You must first respect yourself, and then you must respect the game. What you have read in this book has been proven effective. So you don't have to do no guinea-pig mackin'. There is no need for you to experiment with your game by making mistakes that many macks have made long before you even came on the scene. Hopefully, this book will save you from years of mistakes that men have commonly made when it comes to dating. All you have to do is follow what you've learned here, and everything else will fall into place.

Remember to Keep Up Your Standards

As a mack, do not accept lackluster females. A mack's game naturally elevates. In a true mack's life, the next female is always better than the last. Focus on stacking your paper, and once your paper is stacked, the same females will still be available and then some.

Never focus all your energy on jockin' one female. Like I said, there are over a million females coming of age every single day. Your game is going to be compatible with at least one of these females. Like I said before, the dating game is always something of a gamble. But even if you're in Las Vegas, you should never spend too much time in one casino. If you aren't winning at the MGM Grand, you might need to go over to the Mandalay Bay and try your luck there. The same goes with dating. If your game isn't working with one female, don't waste time wondering why. Don't waste time trying to win her over. Take your game to one of the millions of other females out there who are looking for good game.

Your License to Mack

By reading this book, fully comprehending it, and utilizing its techniques accordingly, you have earned a license to mack. And you must carefully maintain your mack license if you want to have continued success in the game. Here's a list of ten violations that will get your mack license revoked:

1. Spending more than $100 on a first date
2. Allowing a female to disrespect you
3. Having sex with three or more females who rate less than a five (on a scale of one to ten) within a one-month time span
4. Stalking a female
5. Showing up at a female's house with flowers or balloons on a first date
6. Letting a female pit you against another man
7. Calling a female and playing Brian McKnight songs on her voicemail
8. Buying drinks for a female and all her friends at the club
9. Allowing yourself to be pussy-whipped
10. Contemplating suicide because a female hurt you (This is the ultimate mack violation, because a true mack knows his own value)

Be Sure to Maintain a Mack's Demeanor

The majority of this book has been pretty straightforward, but some parts were educational, and some parts were even funny. I wanted this book to create a different range of feelings, because that's part of what the mackin' game is all about. When you're dealing with different females, you need to be able to switch up your demeanor at the drop of the hat.

With some women you have to be serious. With others, you have to take on the demeanor of a teacher and school them on some things. And sometimes you need to be witty. So as a mack, your demeanor needs to be like liquid. It has to be able to flow in any particular direction at any given moment.

My Personal Tastes

People always ask me, "Tariq, what do you look for in women you date?" The answer is: nice feet. If you want to be a true mack, fellas, you have to become a foot reader. In most cases, a woman's feet will tell you everything you need to know about her. The way her feet look will give you an idea about her real age, her income status, whether or not she is going through hard times, etc. Everything else on a woman's body can be camouflaged. Women can use makeup, wigs, breast implants, liposuction, and many other things to camouflage other bodily flaws. But you can't camouflage jacked-up feet. The feet tell the real story. You might meet a woman who fixes up her face and body to *look like* she's twenty-three or twenty-four years old, and she might even *claim* to be twenty-three or twenty-four years old. But if her feet have liver spots, you will be able to peep game and realize that this woman is not what she seems.

I also consider myself a breast man. Most guys are either ass men or breast men. Even though many guys like both (me included), some guys lean toward one end of the spectrum. Now I like nice asses, too, but like I said, if I have to choose, I tend to be more of a breast man.

You'll notice that the more money a man makes, the more of a breast man he becomes. Because of easy access to breast augmentation, a female with nice breasts can maintain her overall looks much longer than a female with a nice ass. She's got to manually maintain that ass. And most women don't have the discipline to go to the gym every day to keep their asses intact.

Top Five Celebrity Females I Would Consider My Type

1. Halle Berry
2. Christina Milian
3. Jessica Alba
4. Mya
5. Mariah Carey (A lot of people may criticize me for giving props to Mariah, but I think there's something sexy about her crazy ass.)

And just to show that I don't discriminate, here's a list of females over the age of forty-five who I think are still "doable":

Top Five Celebrity Females over the Age of Forty-five I Would Consider My Type

1. Sheryl Lee Ralph
2. Beverly Johnson
3. Debbie Allen
4. Angela Bassett
5. Bernadette Stantis (Thelma from *Good Times*)

My Final Piece of Mack Advice

You are either a mack or a trick. Women are either going to bring things to your table, or take things off your table. You are going to be a *player,* or you are going to *pay her.*

A lot of men don't realize this, but most women feel like you owe them something if you have sex with them. Women feel if they have sex with you, they don't have to bring anything else to the table. As a mack, you can't accept this. You have to accept your status as a mack. And **if you accept your mack status, others will accept it, too.**

ABOUT THE AUTHOR

Tariq "King Flex" Nasheed is a fomer hustler and the author of the bestseller *The Art of Mackin'* and *Play or Be Played*. He lives in Los Angeles, and you can find him online at www.kingflex.tv.

Printed in the United States
by Baker & Taylor Publisher Services